# ONE STOP DOC

# Gastroenterology
# and Renal Medicine

D1380078

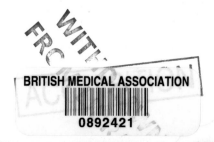

## One Stop Doc

**Titles in the series include:**

Cardiovascular System – Jonathan Aron
Editorial Advisor – Jeremy Ward

Cell and Molecular Biology – Desikan Rangarajan and David Shaw
Editorial Advisor – Barbara Moreland

Endocrine and Reproductive Systems – Caroline Jewels and Alexandra Tillett
Editorial Advisor – Stuart Milligan

Gastrointestinal System – Miruna Canagaratnam
Editorial Advisor – Richard Naftalin

Musculoskeletal System – Bassel Zebian and Wayne Lam
Editorial Advisor – Alistair Hunter

Nervous System – Elliott Smock
Editorial Advisor – Clive Coen

Nutrition and Metabolism – Miruna Canagaratnam and David Shaw
Editorial Advisors – Barbara Moreland and Richard Naftalin

Respiratory System – Jo Dartnell and Michelle Ramsay
Editorial Advisor – John Rees

Renal and Urinary System and Electrolyte Balance – Panos Stamoulos and Spyridon Bakalis
Editorial Advisors – Alistair Hunter and Richard Naftalin

Statistics and Epidemiology – Emily Ferenczi and Nina Muirhead
Editorial Advisor – Lucy Carpenter

Immunology – Stephen Boag and Amy Sadler
Editorial Advisor – John Stewart

Cardiology – Rishi Aggarwal, Emily Ferenczi and Nina Muirhead
Editorial Advisor – Darrel Francis
Volume Editor – Basant Puri

# ONE STOP DOC

# Gastroenterology and Renal Medicine

**Reena Popat** MBBS BSc(Hons)
Senior House Officer in Medicine, Hammersmith Hospital, London, UK

**Danielle Adebayo** MBBS BSc(Hons)
Senior House Officer in Medicine, Hammersmith Hospital, London, UK

**Contributing Author: Thomas Chapman** MBBS BSc(Hons)
Foundation Year 1, Guy's and St Thomas' NHS Trust, London, UK

**Editorial Advisor: Stephen Pereira** BSc(Hons) PhD FRCP
Senior Lecturer in Hepatology & Gastroenterology, The UCL Institute of Hepatology, London, UK

**Volume Editor: Basant Puri** MA PhD MB BChir BSc(Hons) MathSci MRCPsych DipStat MMath
Professor and Consultant in Imaging and Psychiatry and Head of the Lipid Neuroscience Group,
Hammersmith Hospital, London, UK

**Series Editor: Elliott Smock** MBBS BSc(Hons)
Senior House Officer (FY2), University Hospital Lewisham, Lewisham, UK

Hodder Arnold

A MEMBER OF THE HODDER HEADLINE GROUP

First published in Great Britain in 2007 by
Hodder Arnold, an imprint of Hodder Education and a member of the Hodder Headline Group,
an Hachette Livre UK Company, 338 Euston Road, London NW1 3BH

**http://www.hoddereducation.com**

© 2007 Edward Arnold (Publishers) Ltd

Whilst the advice and information in this book are believed to be true and
accurate at the date of going to press, neither the authors nor the publisher
can accept any legal responsibility or liability for any errors or omissions
that may be made. In particular, (but without limiting the generality of the
preceding disclaimer) every effort has been made to check drug dosages;
however it is still possible that errors have been missed. Furthermore,
dosage schedules are constantly being revised and new side-effects
recognized. For these reasons the reader is strongly urged to consult the
drug companies' printed instructions before administering any of the drugs
recommended in this book.

Hodder Headline's policy is to use papers that are natural, renewable and
recyclable products and made from wood grown in sustainable forests.
The logging and manufacturing processes are expected to conform to the
environmental regulations of the country of origin.

*British Library Cataloguing in Publication Data*
A catalogue record for this book is available from the British Library

*Library of Congress Cataloging-in-Publication Data*
A catalog record for this book is available from the Library of Congress

ISBN 978 0340 92556 0

1 2 3 4 5 6 7 8 9 10

Commissioning Editor: Sara Purdy
Project Editor:          Jane Tod
Production Controller: Lindsay Smith
Cover Design:          Amina Dudhia
Indexer:                Indexing Specialists (UK) Ltd

Typeset in 10/12pt Adobe Garamond/Akzidenz GroteskBE by Servis Filmsetting Ltd, Manchester
Printed and bound in Spain

What do you think about this book? Or any other Hodder Arnold title?
Please visit our website at **www.hoddereducation.com**

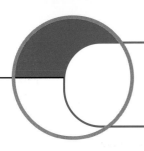

# CONTENTS

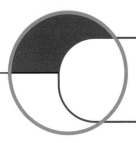

# PREFACE

From the Series Editor, Elliott Smock

Are you ready to face your looming exams? If you have done loads of work, then congratulations; we hope this opportunity to practise SAQs, EMQs, MCQs and Problem-based Questions on every part of the core curriculum will help you consolidate what you've learnt and improve your exam technique. If you don't feel ready, don't panic – the One Stop Doc series has all the answers you need to catch up and pass.

There are only a limited number of questions an examiner can throw at a beleaguered student and this text can turn that to your advantage. By getting straight into the heart of the core questions that come up year after year and by giving you the model answers you need this book will arm you with the knowledge to succeed in your exams. Broken down into logical sections, you can learn all the important facts you need to pass without having to wade through tons of different textbooks when you simply don't have the time. All questions presented here are 'core'; those of the highest importance have been highlighted to allow even shaper focus if time for revision is running out. In addition, to allow you to organize your revision efficiently, questions have been grouped by topic, with answers supported by detailed integrated explanations.

On behalf of all the One Stop Doc authors I wish you the very best of luck in your exams and hope these books serve you well!

From the Authors, Reena Popat and
Danielle Adebayo

This book is intended primarily for clinical medical students preparing for exams in renal medicine and gastroenterology, but will also be useful for junior doctors who are revising. It is not meant to be a textbook of medicine, but highlights key areas often focused on during the exams and in day-to-day clinical practice. We have tried to distil the core topics in this specialty. The questions at the beginning of each topic should help hone in the essential points.

We hope that this book also helps you work through clinical scenarios in a systematic manner, and to develop differential diagnoses and a competent management plan both as clinical students and junior doctors.

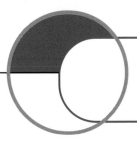

# ABBREVIATIONS

| | |
|---|---|
| AAT | $\alpha_1$-antitrypsin |
| ACE | angiotensin-converting enzyme |
| ACTH | adrenocorticotrophic hormone |
| ADH | antidiuretic hormone |
| AFB | acid-fast bacilli |
| AFP | $\alpha$-fetoprotein |
| Ag | antigen |
| AJCC TNM | American Joint Committee on Cancer, Tumor, Node and Metastases |
| ALF | acute liver failure |
| ALP | alkaline phosphatase |
| ALT | alanine transaminase |
| AMA | antimitochondrial antibody |
| ANA | antinuclear antibody |
| ANCA | antineutrophil cytoplasmic antibody |
| APACHE | Acute Physiology And Chronic Health Evaluation |
| ARDS | acute respiratory distress syndrome |
| ARF | acute renal failure |
| ASO | antistreptolysin O |
| AST | aspartate transaminase |
| ATN | acute tubular necrosis |
| ATP | adenosine triphosphate |
| BDG | bilirubin diglucuronide |
| BE | base excess |
| BM | blood sugar |
| BMG | bilirubin monoglucuronide |
| BP | blood pressure |
| CEA | carcinoembryonic antigen |
| CLF | chronic liver failure |
| CMV | cytomegalovirus |
| CNS | central nervous system |
| CO | cardiac output |
| COPD | chronic obstructive pulmonary disease |
| CRF | chronic renal failure |
| CRP | C-reactive protein |
| Cr | creatinine |
| CRF | chronic renal failure |
| CT | computed tomography |
| CVA | cerebrovascular accident |

| | |
|---|---|
| CVP | central venous pressure |
| DIC | disseminated intravascular coagulation |
| DMSA | dimercaptosuccinic acid |
| DNA | deoxyribonucleic acid |
| dsDNA | double-stranded deoxyribonucleic acid |
| EBV | Epstein–Barr virus |
| ECF | extracellular fluid |
| ECG | electrocardiogram |
| ESR | erythrocyte sedimentation rate |
| ESRF | end-stage renal failure |
| ERCP | endoscopic retrograde cholangiopancreatography |
| FAP | familial adenomatous polyposis |
| FBC | full blood count |
| $F_{IO_2}$ | fraction of inspired oxygen |
| FSGS | focal segmental glomerulosclerosis |
| GBM | glomerular basement membrane |
| GCS | Glasgow coma scale |
| GI | gastrointestinal |
| GFR | glomerular filtration rate |
| GGT | $\gamma$-glutamyl transferase |
| GORD | gastro-oesophageal reflux disease |
| GP | general practitioner |
| Hb | haemoglobin |
| HB | hepatitis B |
| HCC | hepatocellular carcinoma |
| HDU | high-dependency unit |
| 5-HIAA | 5-hydroxy indole-acetic acid |
| HIV | human immunodeficiency virus |
| HLA | human leucocyte antigen |
| HMG CoA | 5-hydroxy-3-methylglutaryl-coenzyme A |
| HNPCC | hereditary non-polyposis colon cancer |
| HR | heart rate |
| HSP | Henoch–Schönlein purpura |
| 5-HT | 5-hydroxytryptamine |
| HUS | haemolytic uraemic syndrome |
| IBD | inflammatory bowel disease |
| IBS | irritable bowel syndrome |
| Ig | immunoglobulin |

| | | | |
|---|---|---|---|
| ITU | intensive therapy unit | PVR | peripheral vascular resistance |
| IV | intravenous | RBC | red blood cell |
| JVP | jugular venous pressure | RF | renal failure |
| KUB | kidneys, ureters and bladder | RNA | ribonucleic acid |
| LDH | lactate dehydrogenase | RUQ | right upper quadrant |
| LMP | last menstrual period | sBP | systolic blood pressure |
| LOS | lower oesophageal sphincter | SCC | squamous cell carcinoma |
| MALT | mucosa-associated lymphoid tissue | SIADH | syndrome of inappropriate ADH secretion |
| MC&S | microscopy, culture and sensitivity | | |
| MEN | multiple endocrine neoplasia | SLE | systemic lupus erythematosus |
| MIBG | $^{131}$iodine-meta-iodobenzylguanidine | TB | tuberculosis |
| MRA | magnetic resonance angiogram | TBW | total body water |
| MRCP | magnetic resonance cholangiopancreatography | TCC | transitional cell carcinoma |
| | | TENS | transcutaneous electrical nerve stimulation |
| MRI | magnetic resonance imaging | | |
| MSU | midstream urine | TIPS | transjugular intrahepatic portosystemic shunt |
| NG | nasogastric tube | | |
| NSAID | non-steroidal anti-inflammatory drug | TNM | tumour, node, metastasis |
| OGD | oesophago-gastroduodenoscopy | TPN | total parenteral nutrition |
| Paco$_2$ | partial pressure of arterial carbon dioxide | TURP | trans-urethral resection of the prostate |
| | | UDP | uridine diphosphate |
| Pao$_2$ | partial pressure of arterial oxygen | UGT | UDP glucuronyl transferase |
| PAS | periodic acid–Schiff | UTI | urinary tract infection |
| PBC | primary biliary cirrhosis | VIP | vasoactive intestinal peptide |
| PET | positron emission tomography | WCC | white cell count |
| PPI | proton pump inhibitor | WHO | World Health Organization |
| PSC | primary sclerosing cholangitis | | |
| PTC | percutaneous transhepatic cholangiography | | |

# SECTION 1

# RENAL MEDICINE

# 1 RENAL MEDICINE

1. For the following scenarios choose the most appropriate fluid replacement. Each option may be used once only

**Options**

A. Normal saline
B. Dextrose saline
C. Normal saline + 20 mmol KCl
D. Normal saline + 80 mmol KCl
E. Albumin

F. Blood
G. Gelofusin
H. 5 per cent dextrose
I. Hartmann's solution
J. 1.26 per cent sodium bicarbonate

1. A 73-year-old patient with confusion, a pulsatile abdominal mass, heart rate of 144 bpm, blood pressure of 84/56 mmHg and anuria
2. A 35-year-old patient presenting with vomiting and diarrhoea, tachycardia and postural hypotension
3. A 20-year-old patient with the first presentation of type 1 diabetes mellitus presenting with diabetic ketoacidosis on an insulin sliding scale and a blood sugar (BM) of 7.8 mmol/L
4. A 78-year-old woman with confusion, plasma $Na^+$ of 168 mmol/L and $K^+$ of 4.2 mmol/L
5. A 40-year-old patient admitted with pyelonephritis, now has oliguria and reduced CVP

2. Typical fluid volumes in a 70 kg man are

**Options**

A. 42 L
B. 60 L
C. 3.5 L
D. 7.5 L
E. 18 L
F. 28 L
G. 10.5 L
H. 5.5 L
I. 14 L
J. 25 L

1. Total body water
2. Intracellular
3. Extracellular
4. Interstitial
5. Intravascular

3. When assessing a patient's hydration status, the following are signs of mild dehydration

a. Oliguria
b. Reduced skin turgor
c. Confusion

d. Compromised cardiovascular status
e. Dry mucous membranes

BM, blood sugar; CVP, central venous pressure; ECF, extracellular fluid

## EXPLANATION: FLUID AND ELECTROLYTE BALANCE

The nephron and extra-renal mechanisms play a vital role in body fluid and electrolyte homeostasis. The fluid compartments in a 70 kg man can be demonstrated as below:

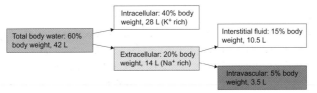

Water moves freely between these compartments with changes in osmolality. The principal cation in the extracellular fluid (ECF) is $Na^+$, which is the major indicator of plasma osmolality.

$$\text{Plasma osmolality} = 2\{[Na^+]+[K^+]\}+\text{blood [glucose]}+\text{blood [urea]}$$

### FLUID LOSS
- Sensible: renal = 1500 mL + gastrointestinal = 100 mL
- Insensible: skin = 500 mL + respiratory = 400 mL.

### FLUID INTAKE
Ingested = 2100 mL + metabolic = 400 mL.

Adults require 30–35 mL/kg/day of water, 2 mmol/kg/day $Na^+$ and 0.5–1 mmol/kg/day $K^+$ for maintenance of normal fluid and electrolyte balance. Abnormal losses of fluids and electrolytes can be secondary to vomiting, diarrhoea, the polyuric phase of renal failure and burns. Fluids administered in the clinical setting can be divided into:
- **Crystalloids**: it is important to know the major constituents of crystalloids administered on the wards:

| Solution | $Na^+$ (mmol/L) | $Cl^-$ (mmol/L) | $K^+$ (mmol/L) | Other (mmol/L) | Osmolality (mosmol/L) |
|---|---|---|---|---|---|
| Normal saline | 154 | 154 | – | – | 308 |
| 0.45% saline | 77 | 77 | – | – | 154 |
| 5% dextrose | – | – | – | – | 278 |
| Hartmann's solution | 131 | 112 | 5 | $HCO_3^-$ 29, $Ca^{2+}$ 4 | 281 |
| Dextrose saline | 31 | 31 | – | – | 284 |

It is safe to administer $K^+$ when the urine output is >40 mL/h. It should not be administered faster than 40 mmol/h, and no greater than 40 mmol of $K^+$ should be added to a 1 L fluid bag.
- **Colloids** such as gelofusin, human albumin solution, human plasma protein fraction and dextran.
- **Blood and blood products**.

When assessing a patient's hydration status, a thorough history, examination and a fluid balance chart of input and output is essential. **Mild** dehydration (<4 per cent body weight loss) is characterized by thirst, reduced skin turgor, sunken eyes and dry mucous membranes. Features of **moderate** dehydration (4–8 per cent body weight loss) include oliguria, orthostatic hypotension, tachycardia and reduced CVP (normal 3–8 cmH₂O). Patients with **severe** dehydration (8–10 per cent body weight loss) present with profound oliguria, a compromised cardiovascular status and confusion.

### Answers
**1.** 1 – F, 2 – C, 3 – H, 4 – A, 5 – G
**2.** 1 – A, 2 – F, 3 – I, 4 – G, 5 – C
**3.** F T F F T

**4.** You are the admitting doctor in the emergency department. An 84-year-old woman is brought by ambulance, having been found collapsed at home. She presents with oliguria, dry mucous membranes, confusion and convulsions

    **a.** The patient's blood results come back from the laboratory, and the serum sodium is 165 mmol/L. What is the normal range of plasma $[Na^+]$?

    **b.** What are the possible causes of this patient's hypernatraemia? What is the most likely cause in this case?

    **c.** How would you manage this patient initially?

    **d.** Describe how you would investigate this patient

**5.** Possible investigations for hypernatraemia include

    **a.** Blood glucose levels

    **b.** Urea and creatinine levels

    **c.** Blood cortisol levels

    **d.** Spinal MRI

    **e.** Added water deprivation test

## EXPLANATION: SODIUM BALANCE

The normal range of plasma [Na$^+$] is 135–145 mmol/L **(4a)**. Refer to the Appendix, page 151 for the physiological mechanisms controling Na$^+$ homeostasis.

### HYPERNATRAEMIA ([Na$^+$] >150 mmol/L)

The patient can present with pyrexia, nausea and vomiting, signs and symptoms of dehydration, convulsions, focal neurology and coma.

Causes are identified below **(4b)**:

|  | **Extra-renal** | **Renal** |
|---|---|---|
| Pure water depletion | Failure of water intake (elderly, post-operatively)<br>Fever<br>Hyperventilation<br>Adipsia (anterior communicating artery aneurysm,<br>   intra-hypothalamic or pituitary haemorrhage,<br>   neoplasm, granuloma) | Diabetes insipidus<br>Chronic renal failure |
| Hypotonic fluid loss | Diarrhoea<br>Vomiting<br>Excessive sweating | Osmotic diuresis, e.g.<br>diabetes mellitus, excess urea<br>Mannitol use |
| Salt gain | Iatrogenic (IV fluids, antibiotics in Na$^+$ salt solutions)<br>Cushing's syndrome<br>Conn's syndrome ($\uparrow$BP, $\uparrow$K$^+$, $\uparrow$HCO$_3^-$) | |

Possible investigations include **(4d)**:
- Urine osmolality and [Na$^+$]. Added water deprivation test:
  - high urine output and osmolality – osmotic diuresis
  - urine osmolality < plasma osmolality – suggests diabetes insipidus
- Blood glucose, renal profile ([Na$^+$], [K$^+$], urea and Cr levels)
- Blood cortisol levels
- Head CT/MRI to exclude a pituitary tumour.

The rehydration must **be gradual over 48 to 72 h (4c)** to prevent the risk of cerebral oedema. The fluid of choice is often normal saline (relatively hypotonic in hypernatraemia). Correct [Na$^+$] at a rate of <0.5 mmol/L/h. The underlying cause should also be addressed.

Continued on page 7

Answers

**4.** See explanation. The most likely cause is dehydration
**5.** T T T F T

## 6. Causes of hyponatraemia include

    **a.** Diabetes insipidus
    **b.** Addison's disease
    **c.** Hypothyroidism
    **d.** Conn's syndrome
    **e.** Subarachnoid haemorrhage

## 7. Hyponatraemia may present with

    **a.** Pyrexia
    **b.** Coma
    **c.** Convulsions
    **d.** Vomiting
    **e.** Dehydration

ADH, antidiuretic hormone; IV, intravenous; SIADH, syndrome of inappropriate ADH secretion; TURP, trans-urethral resection of the prostate

## EXPLANATION: SODIUM BALANCE  Cont'd from page 5

### HYPONATRAEMIA ([Na⁺] <130 mmol/L)

This is more common than hypernatraemia. The patient can present with nausea and vomiting, lethargy, muscle weakness, confusion, ataxia, convulsions and coma.

Causes include:

**Eutonic:**
- Pseudohyponatraemia – hyperglycaemia, hyperlipidaemia
- Surgical irrigation fluids (TURP syndrome)

**Hypotonic:**
- Hypovolaemia:
  - diuretic use
  - Addison's disease
  - renal tubular acidosis
  - diarrhoea
  - vomiting
  - subarachnoid haemorrhage
- Normovolaemia:
  - SIADH
  - iatrogenic: IV fluids; paracetamol and indometacin (potentiate ADH at collecting tubule); barbiturates, opioids, carbamazepine and tricyclics (increase ADH secretion)
  - hypothyroidism
  - renal failure
  - pseudohyponatraemia
- Hypervolaemia:
  - congestive heart failure
  - cirrhosis
  - nephrotic syndrome.

Possible investigations include:
- Urine osmolality and [Na⁺]. The latter will help differentiate renal from non-renal causes
- Blood glucose, renal profile, lipid profile, thyroid profile and cortisol level
- Imaging studies depending on the cause, for example, chest X-ray for heart failure.

**Acute hyponatraemia** (<48 h duration) with the presence of neurological symptoms should be **corrected quickly** using hypertonic 3 per cent saline, which can be combined with loop diuretics to increase water excretion. **Chronic hyponatraemia** (>48 h duration) should be **corrected gradually to prevent central pontine myelinolysis**. The underlying cause should be treated. Patients with hypervolaemic or normovolaemic hypotonic hyponatraemia may need to be fluid restricted and the underlying cause should be treated.

Answers

**6.** F T T F T
**7.** T T T T T

## 8. Regarding hyperkalaemia

a.  It can present with paralytic ileus
b.  It is associated with acidosis
c.  ECG changes include peaked T waves and narrowed QRS complexes
d.  IV calcium gluconate is used to reduce blood $K^+$ levels
e.  ECG changes can progress to asystole if left untreated

## 9. ECG changes associated with hyperkalaemia include

a.  Tall peaked T waves
b.  Shortened QT interval
c.  Widened QRS complex
d.  Widened P waves
e.  Ventricular fibrillation

## 10. As the on-call junior doctor on Saturday night, you are called to see a 27-year-old patient with chronic renal failure whose latest biochemistry results have demonstrated a serum potassium of 7 mmol/L. You note that his last venesection was performed by an inexperienced phlebotomist using a needle and syringe

a.  What is the normal range of plasma $[K^+]$?
b.  Describe the common causes of hyperkalaemia. What are two possible causes of this patient's biochemistry result?
c.  You take an arterial blood gas sample that provides an instant serum potassium level of 7.2 mmol/L. What is this patient at risk of?
d.  How would you manage this patient initially?

## 11. Regarding hypokalaemia

a.  ECG changes include ST segment elevation and a widened QRS complex
b.  It can present with generalized muscle weakness
c.  It is most commonly the result of insufficient dietary intake
d.  It can occur as part of refeeding syndrome
e.  It may be associated with hypomagnesaemia

---

ECG, electrocardiogram; GI, gastrointestinal; IV, intravenous

## EXPLANATION: POTASSIUM BALANCE

The normal range of plasma $[K^+]$ is 3.5–5 mmol/L **(10a)**.

HYPERKALAEMIA ($[K^+]$ >5 mmol/L)
The clinical features of hyperkalaemia include:
- Muscle weakness
- ECG changes (see figure opposite): tall peaked T waves, shortened QT interval, widened QRS complex, widening and eventually loss of P waves, sine wave pattern, ventricular fibrillation.

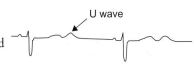
Tall peaked T waves

Widened QRS complex

Aetiology is as follows **(10b)**:
- **Pseudohyperkalaemia**: prolonged tourniquet use, *in vitro* haemolysis, delayed transfer of sample for analysis and hyperventilation
- **Excessive intake**: blood transfusion and excessive IV infusion
- **Impaired excretion**: renal failure, Addison's disease and drugs such as $K^+$-sparing diuretics
- **Tissue redistribution**: trauma, burns, rhabdomyolysis, tumour lysis syndrome, haemolysis and acidosis.

$[K^+]$>6.5 mmol/L is an emergency and requires prompt treatment as it can lead to sudden death from cardiac arrhythmias **(10c)**.

EMERGENCY MANAGEMENT OF HYPERKALAEMIA **(10d)**:
**Immediate**:
- To protect myocardium: 10 mL 10 per cent calcium gluconate IV if ECG changes (may be repeated every 10 min until ECG normalizes)
- To lower serum potassium: insulin (Actrapid 10 units) and 50 mL 20 per cent dextrose IV; nebulized salbutamol (5–10 mg) to drive $K^+$ intracellularly.

**Longer term**:
- To deplete body $K^+$: polysterene sulphonate resins – 30 g enema; 15 g orally three times daily.
Consider need for dialysis.

HYPOKALAEMIA ($[K^+]$ <3.5 mmol/L)
The clinical features of hypokalaemia include:
- Anorexia, nausea, muscle weakness, paralytic ileus
- ECG changes (see figure opposite): small or inverted T waves, increased height of U wave, ST segment depression, widened QRS complex.

U wave

Aetiology is as follows:
- **Increased GI loss**: diarrhoea, vomiting, fistulae, villous adenoma, refeeding syndrome and laxatives
- **Increased renal loss**: diuretics, hyperaldosteronism, renal artery stenosis and osmotic diuresis
- **Tissue redistribution**: insulin therapy, alkalosis and catecholamines
- **Reduced intake** (rare).

Hypokalaemia can be associated with hypomagnesaemia, therefore magnesium deficiency must be sought and corrected first.

Answers
**8.** F T F F T
**9.** T T T T T
**10.** See explanation
**11.** F T F T T

## 12. Concerning metabolic acidosis

    **a.** The pH of plasma is increased
    **b.** Causes can be differentiated by calculating the anion gap
    **c.** If chronic, it leads to an increase in the $Paco_2$
    **d.** It can result after severe haemorrhage
    **e.** Salicylate poisoning always results in metabolic acidosis

## 13. A 30-year-old patient presents with pH 7.2, $Paco_2$ 3.0 kPa, base excess −7, $HCO_3^-$ 17 mmol/L, $Na^+$ 136 mmol/L, $K^+$ 4.2 mmol/L, $Cl^-$ 108 mmol/L. The possible causes of this picture include

    **a.** Ileostomy                   **d.** Methanol ingestion
    **b.** Diabetic ketoacidosis       **e.** Uraemia
    **c.** Renal tubular acidosis

## EXPLANATION: ACID–BASE BALANCE

Acid–base disturbances are commonly associated with renal impairment. However, they may also follow respiratory pathologies. Differentiation between metabolic and respiratory disturbances can be determined by measuring the parameters of acid–base status.

**Normal acid–base** values are as follows:
- pH 7.35–7.45
- $Pao_2$ 10.5–14 kPa
- $Paco_2$ 4.5–6 kPa
- $HCO_3^-$ 22–26 mmol/L
- BE ±2 mmol/L.

| | pH | $Paco_2$ | $HCO_3^-$ |
|---|---|---|---|
| Metabolic acidosis | ↓ | ↔/↓ | ↓ |
| Metabolic alkalosis | ↑ | ↔/↑ | ↑ |
| Respiratory acidosis | ↓ | ↑ | ↔/↑ |
| Respiratory alkalosis | ↑ | ↓ | ↔/↓ |

Causes of **metabolic acidosis** include:
- **Normal anion gap** $(10-18$ mmol/L$=([Na^+]+[K^+])-([Cl^-]+[HCO_3^-]))$; this signifies $HCO_3^-$ loss):
  - diarrhoea
  - biliary/pancreatic fistulae
  - ileostomy
  - renal tubular acidosis
  - Addison's disease
  - hyperalimentation (TPN)
- **High anion gap** ($>18$ mmol/L, suggests the presence of abnormal acid production):
  - diabetic ketoacidosis
  - lactic acidosis
  - renal failure
  - salicylate intoxication
  - methanol or ethylene glycol ingestion
  - paraldehyde poisoning
  - inborn errors of metabolism, e.g. HMG CoA lyase deficiency.

Metabolic acidosis is often partially compensated for by hyperventilation (reduced $Paco_2$).

The underlying cause should be treated. In life-threatening cases (pH $<7.2$), sodium bicarbonate can be infused slowly.

Continued on page 13

Answers
**12.** F T F T F
**13.** T F T F F

### 14. Concerning respiratory acidosis

**a.** It is associated with a bounding pulse
**b.** It can occur in patients with Guillain–Barré syndrome
**c.** It may result from opiate overdose
**d.** Renal retention of bicarbonate may occur in chronic cases
**e.** Treatment may include respiratory support

### 15. For the following blood gases choose the most appropriate diagnosis. Each option may be used once only

**Options**

**A.** Diarrhoea
**B.** Vomiting
**C.** Hyperventilation
**D.** Salicylate intoxication
**E.** Acute COPD exacerbation

**F.** COPD patient treated with 60 per cent $O_2$
**G.** Chronic COPD
**I.** Altitude
**H.** Normal
**J.** Diabetic ketoacidosis

**1.** pH 7.25, $PaCO_2$ 7.8 kPa, $PaO_2$ 8.5 kPa, $HCO_3^-$ 25 mmol/L
**2.** pH 7.37, $PaCO_2$ 8.1 kPa, $PaO_2$ 7.8 kPa, $HCO_3^-$ 35 mmol/L
**3.** pH 7.5, $PaCO_2$ 3 kPa, $PaO_2$ 13.5 kPa, $HCO_3^-$ 24 mmol/L
**4.** pH 7.22, $PaCO_2$ 2.8 kPa, $PaO_2$ 11 kPa, $HCO_3^-$ 18 mmol/L
**5.** pH 7.49, $PaCO_2$ 4.1 kPa, $PaO_2$ 11 kPa, $HCO_3^-$ 30 mmol/L

ARDS, acute respiratory distress syndrome; CNS, central nervous system; COPD, chronic obstructive pulmonary disease; CVA, cerebrovascular accident; NG, nasogastric tube; $PaCO_2$, partial pressure of arterial carbon dioxide; $PaO_2$, partial pressure of arterial oxygen

## EXPLANATION: ACID–BASE BALANCE Cont'd from page 11

Causes of **metabolic alkalosis** include:
- **Loss of acid:**
  - vomiting
  - NG suction
  - gastrocolic fistula
  - hyperaldosteronism
  - diuretic use
- **Gain of $HCO_3^-$:**
  - sepsis
  - exogenous alkali, e.g. antacid abuse
  - over-treatment of acidosis.

Metabolic alkalosis is rarely partially compensated for by hypoventilation, as the associated reduction in $PaO_2$ stimulates the respiratory centres. The underlying cause should be treated.

Causes of **respiratory acidosis** include:
- **Respiratory depression**: central causes such as CVA, drug overdose, e.g. opiates and late salicylate poisoning
- **Muscular weakness**: Guillain–Barré syndrome, myasthenia gravis, botulinum poisoning
- **Infection**: pneumonia
- **Acute respiratory diseases**: asthma, acute exacerbation of COPD.

Signs of $CO_2$ retention may occur. These include bounding pulse, flap tremor and papilloedema.

Chronic cases of respiratory acidosis may be partially compensated for by renal retention of $HCO_3^-$ (metabolic alkalosis). Treatment involves management of the underlying cause, and may include ventilatory support.

Causes of **respiratory alkalosis** include:
- CNS lesions (CVA), neoplasm, infection
- Salicylate intoxication
- Septicaemia
- Anxiety
- High altitude
- Cirrhosis
- Pneumonia
- Pulmonary embolus
- ARDS
- Pulmonary oedema.

Chronic cases of respiratory alkalosis may be partially compensated for by increased renal excretion of $HCO_3^-$ (metabolic acidosis). The underlying cause should be addressed.

Answers
**14.** T T T T T
**15.** 1 – E, 2 – G, 3 – C, 4 – J, 5 – B

### 16. The following are causes of acute renal failure

a. Hypovolaemia
b. Sepsis
c. Polycystic kidney disease
d. Prostate disease
e. Renovascular disease

### 17. Acute renal failure is associated with

a. Anaemia
b. Hyperkalaemia
c. Hyperphosphataemia
d. Normal renal size
e. Polyuria

### 18. When considering acute tubular necrosis

a. It most often results from renal ischaemia
b. Drugs commonly implicated include NSAIDs and aminoglycosides
c. It is always reversible on reperfusion of the kidney
d. The urine sodium is typically greater than 40 mmol/L
e. The urine osmolality is greater than in pre-renal causes of ARF

### 19. Draw a table differentiating the urinary findings in acute tubular necrosis and pre-renal acute renal failure

---

ARF, acute renal failure; ATN, acute tubular necrosis; Cr, creatinine; GFR, glomerular filtration rate; GI, gastrointestinal; NSAID, non-steroidal anti-inflammatory drug

# EXPLANATION: ACUTE RENAL FAILURE

Acute renal failure (ARF) is defined as a rapid decline in renal function over hours to days that leads to retention of nitrogenous waste products (urea and Cr) and impairment of the acid–base balance. It is usually characterized by oliguria (<400 mL/day), however, 10–15% of cases are non-oliguric. The glomerular filtration rate (GFR) may fall by approximately 50 per cent before blood Cr levels rise, hence blood Cr is not a sensitive measure of ARF.

## PRE-RENAL CAUSES

- **Hypovolaemia**: haemorrhage, GI loss, third space loss (pancreatitis), renal loss (diabetes insipidus), skin and mucous membrane losses (burns)
- **Systemic hypotension**: cardiogenic shock, sepsis and liver failure
- **Renovascular disease**: renal artery stenosis.

## RENAL CAUSES

- **Acute tubular necrosis** (ATN): caused by pre-renal causes and nephrotoxins which include extrinsic (NSAIDs, aminoglycosides, ciclosporin, cisplatin) and intrinsic (haemoglobinuria, myoglobinuria, myeloma light chains) causes. As shown below, ARF and ATN are a continuum.

Pre-renal ARF ⟶ ATN
Reversible on reperfusion    Irreversible on reperfusion

They can be differentiated as shown by the table below **(19)**:

|  | Pre-renal | ATN |
|---|---|---|
| Urine osmolality (mosmol/kg) | >500 | <400 |
| Urine/plasma osmolality | >1.3 | <1.1 |
| Urine/plasma Cr | >40 | <20 |
| Urine Na$^+$ (mmol/L) | <20 | >40 |
| Fractional Na$^+$ excretion (%) | <1 | >1 |

- **Acute interstitial necrosis** (causes as above)
- **Acute cortical necrosis**: seen in placental abruption
- **Small-vessel disease**: vasculitides and malignant hypertension
- **Glomerular disease**.

Continued on page 17

## Answers

**16.** T T F T T
**17.** F T F T F
**18.** T T F T F
**19.** See explanation

**20. Theme – Renal failure investigations. For the following scenarios choose the most appropriate diagnostic investigation. Each option may be used once only**

Options

A. Renal ultrasound
B. Hysterosalpingogram
C. KUB X-ray
D. MRA
E. Renal venogram
F. Cystogram
G. Anti-dsDNA
H. Isotope renogram
I. Creatine kinase level
J. Urine dipstick

1. A 24-year-old African-Caribbean female with polyarthritis, facial rash and proteinuria
2. A 45-year-old female with stage III cervical cancer presenting with oliguria and pruritus
3. A 70-year-old male smoker with ARF following recent commencement of an angiotensin receptor blocker
4. An elderly female, admitted after being discovered by her social worker following a fall, producing dark urine
5. A middle-aged patient with sudden-onset left-sided loin pain radiating to the scrotum, and haematuria

---

ANA, antinuclear antibody; ANCA, antineutrophil cytoplasmic antibody; ARF, acute renal failure; ATN, acute tubular necrosis; CRF, chronic renal failure; dsDNA, double-stranded deoxyribonucleic acid; KUB, kidneys, ureters and bladder; MRA, magnetic resonance angiogram; RBC, red blood cell; SLE, systemic lupus erythematosus

## EXPLANATION: ACUTE RENAL FAILURE Cont'd from page 15

### POST-RENAL CAUSES

|              | Ureteric                                                         | Bladder neck                                                     | Urethral                             |
|--------------|------------------------------------------------------------------|------------------------------------------------------------------|--------------------------------------|
| Extraluminal | Pelvic surgery ligation, cervical cancer, retroperitoneal fibrosis | Prostate disease (benign and malignant)                          | Phimosis                             |
| Intramural   | Post-operative oedema                                            | Bladder cancer, drugs: tricyclics, cystitis with mural oedema    | Stricture: instrumental, infectious  |
| Intraluminal | Stones, blood clots, sloughed renal papillae                    |                                                                  |                                      |

Important investigations in ARF include:
- Urinalysis: red blood cell (RBC) casts are present in glomerulonephritis, vasculitis or malignant hypertension. White cell casts can be noted in pyelonephritis. Epithelial cell casts are present in ATN or glomerulonephritis
- Arterial blood gas
- Full blood count: anaemia is more indicative of chronic renal failure (CRF)
- Renal profile
- Liver profile and hepatitis screen
- Bone profile: hypocalcaemia and hyperphosphataemia is more indicative of CRF
- Autoantibodies: antineutrophil cytoplasmic antibody (ANCA), antinuclear antibody (ANA), anti-dsDNA for ARF aetiology
- Complement level: reduced in systemic lupus erythematosus (SLE) and post-infectious glomerulonephritis
- Myeloma screen: urinary Bence Jones protein, protein electrophoresis, immunoglobulin levels
- Renal ultrasound: to exclude stones, hydronephrosis and tumours. Small kidneys suggest CRF
- Kidneys, ureters and bladder (KUB) X-ray: 80 per cent of renal stones are radio-opaque
- Radionuclide renal scan: exclude obstruction, scarring
- Renal biopsy.

Prevention is by identification of patients at risk. The major causes of death in ARF are **pulmonary oedema** and **hyperkalaemia**. Mortality rates are directly related to the underlying cause of ARF. In general, the mortality remains 50 per cent. Oliguric ARF has a worse prognosis than non-oliguric ARF.

Answer

**20.** 1 – G, 2 – A, 3 – D, 4 – I, 5 – C

## 21. Consider chronic renal failure

**a.** The commonest cause is hypertension
**b.** Adult-onset polycystic kidney disease is associated with hepatic cysts
**c.** Kimmelstiel–Wilson nodular glomerulosclerosis is pathognomonic of hypertensive nephropathy
**d.** Recurrent cystitis is a cause of chronic renal failure
**e.** It can be caused by liver cirrhosis

## 22. Write short notes on the complications of chronic renal failure

## 23. Regarding chronic renal failure

**a.** End-stage renal failure is characterized by a GFR of <30mL/min
**b.** GI bleed is a common complication
**c.** Hyperglycaemia is a complication of peritoneal dialysis
**d.** The hypocalcaemia associated with CRF is partly attributable to hyperphosphataemia
**e.** Pruritus can be a presenting complaint

CRF, chronic renal failure; ESRF, end-stage renal failure; GFR, glomerular filtration rate; GI, gastrointestinal

## EXPLANATION: CHRONIC RENAL FAILURE

Chronic renal failure is defined as **irreversible chronic renal damage resulting in more than 50 per cent loss of renal function**. It can be divided into three main categories: **mild** (GFR 30–70 mL/min), **moderate** (GFR 10–30 mL/min) and **end-stage** (GFR < 10 mL/min, incompatible with survival without renal replacement therapy). In the UK, approximately 80–100/million people/year go on to develop end-stage renal failure (ESRF).

Common causes of CRF include:
- **Diabetic nephropathy** (~40 per cent): associated with hyaline arteriosclerosis, capillary basement membrane thickening, diffuse glomerulosclerosis and pathognomonically Kimmelstiel–Wilson nodular glomerulosclerosis
- **Hypertensive nephroangiosclerosis** (~25 per cent). In malignant hypertension, the kidney has a flea-bitten appearance (petechiae) macroscopically. Histologically, the kidney has an appearance consistent with necrotizing arteriolitis and intimal cellular proliferation producing an 'onion-skinning' effect
- **Glomerulonephritis** (~15 per cent): caused by immune complex deposition with variable histology.

Other causes are polycystic kidney disease, reflux disease, pyelonephritis, obstructive uropathy, vasculitis, multiple myeloma and amyloidosis.

CRF may present with a variety of signs and complications **(22)**:
- **Neurological**: poor memory, apathy, restless legs, proximal myopathy, hyper-reflexia, seizures, asterixis
- **Cutaneous**: pruritus, bruising, yellow skin pigmentation
- **Haematological**: anaemia, bleeding diathesis, infection susceptibility
- **Bone**: osteomalacia, osteoporosis, osteitis fibrosa cystica, hyperparathyroidism
- **Cardiovascular**: pericarditis, hypertension, cardiomyopathy, heart failure, hypercholesterolaemia
- **Respiratory**: pulmonary oedema, pleuritis
- **Gastrointestinal**: anorexia, nausea, vomiting, GI bleed
- **Hypogonadism**: gynaecomastia, impotence, infertility
- **Insulin resistance**.

Continued on page 21

Answers
**21.** F T F F F
**22.** See explanation
**23.** F T T T T

### 24. Management options in chronic renal failure include

a. Desmopressin for bleeding diathesis
b. Statin use
c. Peritoneal dialysis in the obese
d. Calcium carbonate for hyperkalaemia management
e. Spontaneous bacterial peritonitis is a complication of haemodialysis

### 25. Theme – Causes of chronic renal failure. For the following scenarios choose the most appropriate diagnosis. Each option may be used once only

Options

A. Hypertension
B. Systemic sclerosis
C. Diabetes mellitus
D. Wegener's granulomatosis
E. Multiple myeloma

F. Reflux disease
G. Prostate hypertrophy
H. Amyloidosis
I. Microscopic polyangiitis
J. Adult polycystic kidney disease

1. A 42-year-old man presents with haematuria, right-sided flank pain and hypertension. On abdominal examination he has bilateral ballotable masses palpable
2. A 71-year-old woman presents with a fracture of the humerus. The X-ray reveals lytic lesions. Serum protein electrophoresis reveals monoclonal M bands
3. A 48-year-old man presents with peripheral neuropathy, increasing shortness of breath and hypertension. Urine dipstick reveals 3+ protein. Renal biopsy shows apple-green birefringence in polarized light
4. A 39-year-old woman presents with haemoptysis and nasal discharge. A chest X-ray reveals a cavitating lesion. The patient is c-ANCA-positive

ANCA, antineutrophil cytoplasmic antibody; CMV, cytomegalovirus; CRF, chronic renal failure; ESRF, end-stage renal failure; TB, tuberculosis

## EXPLANATION: CHRONIC RENAL FAILURE Cont'd from page 19

Investigations for CRF are the same as those for ARF (see page 17).

Treatment for CRF can be divided into conservative (avoid nephrotoxic drugs, optimize fluid balance, rigorous blood pressure control, iron supplements for anaemia, vitamin D and calcium supplements), dialysis and transplantation. The renal replacement options are highlighted in the box below.

**Dialysis** is a method of waste-product excretion via diffusion and convection from the blood into a dialysis fluid (dialysate) across a semi-permeable membrane. The urgent indications of dialysis include dangerous hyperkalaemia, acidosis, pulmonary oedema or uraemic encephalopathy.

- **Haemodialysis:** prior to haemodialysis, vascular access is achieved by means of a surgically created arterio-venous fistula (synthetic material or use of autologous saphenous vein), double-lumen jugular or femoral catheter. Haemodialysis is performed three times a week. Problems associated with this method of dialysis include: hypotension, dialysis disequilibrium syndrome (an illness associated with over-rapid removal of toxic metabolites ranging from headache to coma), infection, problems with vascular access and amyloidosis.
- **Haemofiltration:** this is well tolerated in acutely ill patients as it can be performed via a central venous catheter, avoids rapid solute changes and there is less probability of haemodynamic instability. However, it is a more expensive method.
- **Peritoneal dialysis:** the peritoneum acts as the semi-permeable membrane. Dialysate is run into the peritoneal cavity via a catheter inserted across the anterior abdominal wall. It is performed four times a day and can be carried out at home. The complications of peritoneal dialysis include: infection, hyperglycaemia and hypertriglyceridaemia, and it is less suitable for obese patients.

**Transplantation** is the ultimate form of treatment for ESRF. Donors are divided into three groups, cadaveric, live related or live non-related. It is crucial to note any history of CMV, herpes zoster and TB as there is a risk of reactivation with immunosuppression post-transplantation. The main classes of drugs used post-transplant include corticosteroids, ciclosporin, azathioprine, antilymphocytic preparations and prophylactic antimicrobials.

The transplant prognosis is directly related to the donor source, cadaveric kidneys fairing worse. The graft survival rate for live donor kidneys is approximately 95 per cent at 1 year and 76 per cent at 5 years, while the graft survival rate for cadaveric kidneys is about 89 per cent at 1 year and 61 per cent at 5 years.

Answers
**24.** T T F F F
**25.** 1– J, 2 – E, 3 – H, 4 – D

## 26. Nephritic syndrome is defined by

a. Proteinuria

b. Hypercholesterolaemia

c. Oedema

d. Haematuria

e. Hypertension

## 27. Regarding glomerulonephritis

a. Changes in minimal change disease are evident at light microscopy

b. Thin basement membrane disease is usually treated with and responds to steroid therapy

c. In IgA nephropathy, haematuria presents 2 days after the infectious episode

d. Membranoproliferative glomerulonephritis responds well to treatment

e. 75 per cent of cases of membranous nephropathy are idiopathic

ESRF, end-stage renal failure; FSGS, focal segmental glomerulosclerosis; GBM, glomerular basement membrane; HIV, human immunodeficiency virus; Ig, immunoglobulin

## EXPLANATION: GLOMERULONEPHRITIS

Glomerulonephritis encompasses renal diseases with an underlying immunological mechanism that triggers inflammatory injury to the glomerulus. The antigen is either exogenous (microbials or drugs) or endogenous (autoimmune process).

It is often defined by renal biopsy findings; other investigations include those for haematuria and proteinuria. The mechanism of injury is either humoral (antibodies, immune complexes, complement) or cellular (T cells, macrophages).

Glomerulonephritis commonly manifests as:
- Proteinuria
- Urinary red cell cast excretion
- Haematuria
- Hypertension
- Peripheral oedema
- Renal failure.

It is referred to as **nephritic syndrome** if the patient presents with oliguria, haematuria, hypertension and oedema.

For simplicity the glomerulonephritides can be divided into the following:

### NORMAL LIGHT MICROSCOPY FINDINGS
- **Minimal change disease**. These patients classically present with nephrotic syndrome. There is fusion of podocyte foot processes at electron microscopy. Peak incidence is in children aged 1–6 years. It usually has a good prognosis and is corticosteroid responsive; 1 per cent progress to ESRF.
- **Thin basement membrane disease** is a benign autosomal dominant condition that affects approximately 3 per cent of the general population and is characterized by extensive glomerular basement membrane (GBM) thinning at electron microscopy. Usually identified incidentally with persistent microscopic haematuria.

### FOCAL GLOMERULAR LESIONS
- **Focal segmental glomerulosclerosis** (FSGS) accounts for about 15 per cent of cases of nephritic syndrome in adults and is characterized by areas of focal scarring. It can be idiopathic or secondary to diseases such as reflux nephropathy and HIV. Management is with steroids.

Continued on page 25

Answers
**26.** F F T T T
**27.** F F T F T

**28. Regarding post-steptococcal glomerulonephritis**

    **a.** It is the most common cause of glomerulonephritis
    **b.** The most commonly affected group are teenage girls
    **c.** Molecular mimicry may be implicated in the pathogenesis
    **d.** A throat swab may be helpful in diagnosis
    **e.** It is associated with a poor prognosis

**29. For the following scenarios choose the most appropriate diagnosis. Each option may be used once only**

**Options**

| | |
|---|---|
| **A.** Membranous nephropathy | **F.** Churg–Strauss syndrome |
| **B.** Post-streptococcal glomerulonephritis | **G.** Goodpasture's syndrome |
| **C.** IgA nephropathy | **H.** Henoch–Schönlein syndrome |
| **D.** Focal segmental glomerulosclerosis | **I.** Thin basement membrane disease |
| **E.** Wegener's granulomatosis | **J.** Minimal change disease |

    **1.** A 7-year-old boy with a skin rash, abdominal pain and per rectal bleed following an upper respiratory tract infection
    **2.** A 6-year-old child with recurrent haematuria following a sore throat with normal C3 and C4 levels
    **3.** Proteinuria in a HIV-positive patient. Renal biopsy shows scarring without increase in cellularity
    **4.** A 24-year-old patient with oedema. Renal biopsy shows normal findings on light microscopy and fusion of podocyte foot processes at electron microscopy
    **5.** An asthmatic patient presenting with haematuria and found to be p-ANCA positive

---

ACE, angiotensin-converting enzyme; ANCA, antineutrophil cytoplasmic antibody; ESRF, end-stage renal failure; GBM, glomerular basement membrane; Ig, immunoglobulin; SLE, systemic lupus erythematosus

## EXPLANATION: GLOMERULONEPHRITIS Cont'd from page 23

### DIFFUSE GLOMERULAR LESIONS

- **IgA nephropathy** is the commonest type of glomerulonephritis and usually occurs in children and young men with intercurrent infections. On microscopy there is diffuse mesangial cell proliferation and mesangium IgA deposition. Approximately 30 per cent progress to ESRF. Patients with no associated hypertension and proteinuria have a better prognosis.
- **Membranous nephropathy** is characterized by increasing thickening of the GBM. Approximately 75 per cent of cases are idiopathic. The remainder are associated with infections such as hepatitis B, drugs (e.g. ACE inhibitors), autoimmune conditions (e.g. diabetes and SLE), neoplasms and post-renal transplantation.
- **Membranoproliferative/mesangiocapillary glomerulonephritis** is characterized by diffuse capillary wall thickening and mesangial cell proliferation. There are three types:
  - **type 1**: characterized by immune deposits along the subendothelial aspects of the GBM. This is the commonest type and is associated with conditions such as SLE and hepatitis B/C
  - **type 2**: there are intramembranous deposits of C3 in the GBM. It is particularly associated with partial lipodystrophy
  - **type 3**: characterized by subendothelial and epimembranous deposits of C3 and IgG.
  Approximately 50 per cent of patients progress to ESRF in 10–15 years.
- **Post-streptococcal glomerulonephritis**. The peak incidence is in 2–6-year-old males, commonly occurring 7–14 days after β-haemolytic streptococcal infection. It is thought that molecular mimicry (antibody to streptococcal antigen cross-reacting with a glomerular antigen) may have a role in pathogenesis. The prognosis is good and <2 per cent of children progress to ESRF.
- **Henoch–Schönlein purpura** usually presents in children under 10 years of age, and is twice as common in males. Manifestations include a purpuric rash on the ankles, dorsum of the legs and buttocks, colicky abdominal pain, fleeting polyarthritis of large joints and microscopic haematuria.
- **Rapidly progressive glomerulonephritis** (crescentic) is characterized by the presence of crescents (epithelial cell proliferation and monocyte accumulation in Bowman's space), which is usually associated with severe renal injury. It can either be primary or associated with systemic disease such as anti-GBM disease, small vessel vasculitis like:
  - Wegener's granulomatosis (c-ANCA positive) – respiratory tract involvement, e.g. sinusitis, nasal bridge collapse, haemoptysis
  - Churg–Strauss syndrome (p-ANCA positive) – associated with asthma and eosinophilia
  - microscopic polyarteritis (p-ANCA positive) – similar to the two above but no granulomatous lesions.
  Treatment options involve the use of cyclophosphamide, corticosteroids and plasma exchange therapy.

Answers
**28.** F F T T F
**29.** 1 – H, 2 – C, 3 – D, 4 – J, 5 – F

## 30. Regarding haematuria

a. Painless macroscopic haematuria is most likely to result from malignancy
b. The presence of haematuria at the end of the urinary stream is indicative of a urethral pathology
c. The presence of red cell casts at cytology suggests glomerulonephritis
d. It can be associated with odynophagia
e. Malaria is a cause of haematuria

## 31. Appropriate initial investigations for the cause of haematuria include

a. Urine cytology
b. IV urogram
c. Renal biopsy
d. Coagulation screen
e. ASO titres

## 32. What are the causes of haematuria?

ASO, antistreptolysin O; HSP, Henoch–Schönlein purpura; Ig, immunoglobulin; IV, intravenous; RBC, red blood cell; SLE, systemic lupus erythematosus; TB, tuberculosis

## EXPLANATION: HAEMATURIA

Haematuria is defined as an abnormal number of red blood cells (RBCs) in the urine. We normally excrete up to $1.2 \times 10^6$ RBC/day (<1 RBC per high-powered field). Haematuria can be divided into:
- **Macroscopic**: gross haematuria, visible to the naked eye
- **Microscopic**: urine appears normal, haematuria is detected on urinalysis.

**Renal causes (32)**:
- Glomerular causes:
  - **proliferative**: IgA nephropathy, HSP, SLE, Goodpasture's syndrome, vasculitis
  - **non-proliferative**: diabetic glomerulosclerosis, Alport's syndrome
- Non-glomerular causes:
  - **trauma**
  - **vascular**: renal infarct, renal vein thrombosis, malignant hypertension
  - **renal neoplasms**
  - **familial**: polycystic kidney syndrome
  - **drug-induced interstitial nephritis.**

**Extra-renal causes (32)**:
- **Calculi**
- **Neoplasia**: bladder, prostate, urethral
- **Infection**: cystitis, prostatitis, urethritis, TB, schistosomiasis
- **Drugs**: anticoagulants, cyclophosphamide (haemorrhagic cystitis)
- **Trauma**
- **Bleeding disorders.**

False causes **(34a)** include menstruation, eating beetroot, drugs (such as rifampicin, phenothiazine and chlor-promazine), haemoglobinuria, myoglobinuria and porphyrins.

Continued on page 29

Answers

**30.** T F T T T
**31.** T F F T T
**32.** See explanation

**33. Choose the most appropriate diagnosis for each of the following scenarios. Each option may be used once only**

**Options**

A. Rheumatic fever
B. Infective endocarditis
C. Calculi
D. Urinary tract infection
E. Goodpasture's syndrome

F. TB
G. Lung cancer
H. Factitious haematuria
I. Bladder cancer
J. Renal cancer

1. A 39-year-old immigrant with gross haematuria after commencing TB treatment
2. A 70-year-old smoker with painless gross haematuria
3. A 24-year-old female with dysuria, frequency and haematuria
4. An IV drug user who presents with fever, night sweats and a new pansystolic murmur
5. A 25-year-old male smoker with haemoptysis, shortness of breath on exertion and haematuria

**34. A 67-year-old female presents to her GP complaining of blood-stained urine**

a. List the common false causes of haematuria
b. What are important questions to ask when taking this patient's history?

CRP, C-reactive protein; ESR, erythrocyte sedimentation rate; FBC, full blood count; GP, general practitioner; HSP, Henoch–Schönlein purpura; HUS, haemolytic uraemic syndrome; IV, intravenous; KUB, kidneys, ureters and bladder; LMP, last menstrual period; MC&S, microscopy, culture and sensitivity; TB, tuberculosis

## EXPLANATION: HAEMATURIA Cont'd from page 27

When taking a history, the following are important factors **(34b)**:
- **Age**: a useful indicator to the aetiology
- **Last menstrual period** (LMP): to exclude contamination of the urine sample
- **Occupation**: industrial carcinogens are a risk factor for renal tract malignancies
- **Symptoms**:
  - onset
  - duration
  - amount
  - timing in the urine stream: initial haematuria suggests a urethral cause, terminal haematuria is suggestive of bladder pathology
  - urinary symptoms: frequency, urgency, dysuria, hesitancy, post-micturation dribble
  - associated symptoms: abdominal pain (cystitis, pyelonephritis, stones, HSP), diarrhoea (HSP, HUS), haemoptysis (TB, vasculitis, Goodpasture's syndrome), fever/night sweats (TB, infective endocarditis), prior odynophagia (post-streptococcal nephropathy), joint pain and swelling (connective tissue diseases, sickle cell disease)
  - past medical history: such as sickle cell disease, urinary congenital abnormalities, valvular heart disease
  - medication: anticoagulation
  - family history: Alport's syndrome, thin basement membrane disease
  - social history: smoking increases the risk of urinary tract malignancy. Include a sexual history (urethritis, prostatitis).

Urine dipstick and MC&S are essential investigations. Red cell casts and dysmorphic RBCs are indicative of glomerular pathology; 24 h urine collection is used to detect the heavy levels of protein needed to make a diagnosis of glomerular disease.

Other investigations include blood analysis (FBC, renal profile, CRP, ESR, coagulation screen, autoantibody screen, prostate specific antigen), KUB X-ray, renal ultrasound, IV urogram, cystoscopy and renal biopsy.

In general, patients above 50 years of age should be referred to a urologist, as the risk of malignancy is high. Patients below 40 years should preferably be referred to a nephrologist, as the cause is more likely to be renal in origin.

Answers

**33.** 1 – H, 2 – I, 3 – D, 4 – B, 5 – E
**34.** See explanation (pages 27 and 29)

### 35. Regarding hypertension

**a.** It is defined by the WHO as a persistently elevated blood pressure above 130/100 mmHg
**b.** It affects up to 30 per cent of the adult population
**c.** Secondary hypertension accounts for the majority of cases
**d.** It is more common in the Asian and African-Caribbean population
**e.** Treatment resistance is suggestive of secondary hypertension

### 36. Risk factors for hypertension include

**a.** Non-insulin-dependent diabetes mellitus
**b.** Family history
**c.** Obesity
**d.** Alcohol
**e.** High salt intake

### 37. Regarding renal artery stenosis

**a.** The commonest cause is fibromuscular dysplasia
**b.** ACE inhibitors are commonly used in the management of secondary hypertension
**c.** It is often associated with other atherosclerotic disease manifestations
**d.** It is noted on ultrasound as a unilateral small kidney
**e.** MRA is the gold standard investigation

### 38. Secondary causes of hypertension: match the clinical scenario with the underlying disorder. Each option may be used once only

**Options**

**A.** Hyperthyroidism
**B.** Dissecting aortic aneurysm
**C.** Coarctation of the aorta
**D.** Essential hypertension
**E.** Conn's syndrome
**F.** Renal artery stenosis
**G.** Renin-producing tumours
**H.** Phaeochromocytoma
**I.** Cushing's syndrome
**J.** Acromegaly

1. A 60-year-old smoker with diabetes mellitus and coronary artery disease, recently started on enalapril, who now has a uraemia and rising blood creatinine
2. A 34-year-old woman with a constantly elevated blood pressure and blood $Na^+$ of 146 mmol/L and $K^+$ of 2.9 mmol/L, which is resistant to normal antihypertensives
3. A middle-aged obese woman, who presents with bruising, striae and hypertension
4. A 25-year-old patient with hypertension, radiofemoral delay on examination and rib notching on the chest X-ray
5. A 17-year-old patient with headaches, palpitations and flushing

ACE, angiotensin-converting enzyme; BP, blood pressure; CO, cardiac output; MRA, magnetic resonance angiogram; PVR, peripheral vascular resistance; WHO, World Health Organization

# EXPLANATION: RENOVASCULAR DISEASE AND HYPERTENSION

Hypertension is defined by the WHO as a **persistently elevated BP above 160/95 mmHg**. Generally BP readings above 140/90 mmHg warrant intervention. The condition affects about 20–30 per cent of the adult population. It is more prevalent in the Asian and African-Caribbean population. The causes of hypertension can be divided into two main groups. **Primary/essential hypertension** accounts for 90 per cent of cases. It is a condition of uncertain aetiology. Multiple factors are thought to contribute to the development of essential hypertension, including genetics and environmental factors (obesity, high alcohol intake, high salt intake and stress). The causes of **secondary hypertension** are summarized below:

| Renal | Endocrine | Others |
|---|---|---|
| Glomerulonephritis | Phaeochromocytoma | Coarctation of the aorta |
| Polycystic kidney disease | Conn's syndrome | Pregnancy |
| Renin-producing tumours | Cushing's syndrome | Oral contraceptive pill |
| Renovascular disease | Hyperthyroidism | |
| | Acromegaly | |

A history of renal disease, young age of onset, treatment resistance and accelerated hypertension are features suggestive of secondary hypertension. Blood pressure is a product of cardiac output (CO) and peripheral vascular resistance (PVR, afterload). The cardiac output is determined by preload, which is affected by body sodium and water handling, as well as contractility. See Appendix, page 151 for the homeostatic mechanisms controlling blood pressure.

Renovascular diseases are a group of disorders characterized by a narrowing of the renal arteries or veins. **Renal artery stenosis** accounts for approximately 50 per cent of all secondary hypertension cases and can occur as a result of atherosclerosis or fibromuscular dysplasia. Unilateral arterial involvement is often associated with hypertension, while involvement of both arteries results in renal failure. Renal artery stenosis results in renal hypoperfusion, which leads to activation of the renin–angiotensin mechanism (see Appendix, page 151).

**Atherosclerotic disease** is the commonest cause of renal artery stenosis. It usually presents in those over the age of 50 years. Affected patients often have other atheromatous disease such as ischaemic heart disease, peripheral vascular disease and cerebrovascular disease. The risk factors are similar to those for other atheromatous disease. The atheromatous lesions are often found proximally around the renal artery ostia, making them amenable to intervention. **Fibromuscular dysplasia** is most often found in young women. The underlying cause of fibromuscular dysplasia is unknown, however smoking, hormonal factors and genetics play a role in the aetiology. The stenosis characteristically affects the distal two-thirds and branches of the renal arteries.

Investigations include: blood sampling (renal profile, renin and aldosterone levels), renal ultrasound (the size of the affected kidney is reduced), duplex ultrasonography, MRA, renal angiography (gold standard investigation).

Management options include cessation of nephrotoxic medication, control of blood pressure and risk factors for atheromatous disease, transluminal angioplasty $\pm$ stent insertion, reconstructive vascular surgery or nephrectomy.

Answers
**35.** F T F T T
**36.** T T T T T
**37.** F F T T F
**38.** 1 – F, 2 – E, 3 – I, 4 – C, 5 – H

## 39. Consider nephrotic syndrome

a. It is characterized by protein excretion >3 g/day
b. It is characterized by hyperalbuminuria
c. There is an increased risk of infection
d. Membranous nephropathy is the commonest cause in children
e. The distinguishing feature on examination is a raised JVP

## 40. An 11-year-old boy presents with nephrotic syndrome; the most appropriate management options include

a. Renal biopsy to determine the underlying cause
b. Steroid therapy
c. Spironolactone
d. High-protein and high-sodium diet
e. Prophylactic heparin therapy

## 41. For the following scenarios choose the most appropriate diagnosis. Each option may be used once only

**Options**

A. Traveller's diarrhoea
B. Acromegaly
C. Amyloidosis
D. Malaria
E. Tuberculosis
F. Methotrexate
G. Penicillamine
H. Minimal change disease
I. Membranous glomerulonephritis
J. Systemic lupus erythematosus

1. A 40-year-old woman presenting with facial oedema after recently starting new medication, with the following findings on examination: ulnar deviation of the fingers, Boutonnière deformity
2. A 24-year-old medical student recently returning from Nigeria with fever, night sweats, mylagia, vomiting and splenomegaly
3. A 45-year-old woman with fatigue, carpal tunnel syndrome, macroglossia, hepatosplenomegaly and nephrotic syndrome. Diagnosis is confirmed by renal biopsy positivity with Congo red staining
4. 36-year-old African-Caribbean woman with peripheral joint arthritis, photosensitive rash, thrombocytopaenia and gross peripheral oedema
5. A 10-year-old boy with periorbital and scrotal oedema. Light microscopy of the renal biopsy specimen reveals no abnormalities

---

ACE, angiotensin-converting enzyme; BP, blood pressure; HIV, human immunodeficiency virus; Ig, immunoglobulin; IV, intravenous; JVP, jugular venous pressure; MC&S, microscopy, culture and sensitivity; RF, renal failure; SLE, systemic lupus erythematosus

## EXPLANATION: PROTEINURIA AND NEPHROTIC SYNDROME

We normally excrete approximately 150 mg protein/day in the urine, due to stringent glomerular filtration via the three-layered glomerular capillary wall and tubular protein reabsorption.

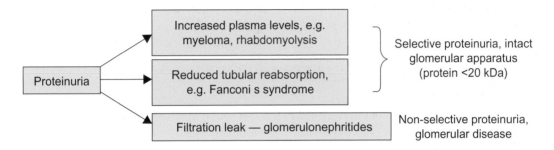

Nephrotic syndrome is characterized by proteinuria >3 g/day, hypoalbuminaemia, oedema and hyperlipidaemia (enhanced hepatic lipid and lipoprotein synthesis). There is also an increased susceptibility to infection as a result of increased IgG and IgA renal loss. Renal excretion of antithrombin produces a hypercoagulable state.

The causes of nephrotic syndrome are:
- Primary glomerulonephritis:
  - **minimal change nephropathy**: commonest cause of nephrotic syndrome. It is characterized by normal light microscopy appearance. Electron microscopy shows widespread fusion of epithelial cell foot processes
  - **membranous nephropathy**: usually idiopathic. Approximately 20 per cent of cases are secondary to infection, drugs, neoplasia and SLE
  - **focal segmental glomerulosclerosis**
  - **mesangiocapillary glomerulonephritis**
- Secondary glomerulonephritis: can be due to diabetes mellitus, amyloidosis, drugs (gold, penicillamine), malignancy, infection (HIV, hepatitis B, malaria), SLE, vasculitis, chronic heart failure and renal vein thrombosis.

Complications of nephrotic syndrome include hypoalbuminaemia, which may cause facial swelling, peripheral oedema, ascites and pleural effusion. Other complications are hyperlipidaemia, hypercoagulability (such as renal vein thrombosis) and acute renal failure due to intravascular volume depletion. Investigations such as urinalysis and MC&S, 24 h urine collection, blood analysis, chest X-ray or renal ultrasound are often required to aid with the diagnosis. Renal biopsy is performed in adults, but usually not in children unless unusual features are present, and in those not responding to steroid therapy.

Management options include: daily weight and BP measurements, low-sodium and high-protein diet (care in RF), strict fluid balance (fluid restriction and, if necessary, IV albumin), treatment of secondary causes, corticosteroid therapy, diuretics (loop diuretics and, if necessary, thiazide diuretics), ACE inhibitors to reduce proteinuria, statins for hyperlipidaemia, anticoagulation in high-risk cases.

Answers
**39.** T T T F F
**40.** F T F F T
**41.** 1 – G, 2 – D, 3 – C, 4 – J, 5 – H

## 42. The following are malignant tumours of the renal tract

a. Renal oncocytoma
b. Renal adenocarcinoma
c. Renal metanephric adenoma
d. Transitional cell carcinoma
e. Nephroblastoma

## 43. Regarding nephroblastoma

a. It is also known as Wilms' tumour
b. It classically occurs in young children
c. Nephroblastomas are purely epithelial in component
d. It is bilateral in 20 per cent of cases
e. It may present with failure to thrive

## 44. A 60-year-old male is referred to urology clinic as his GP is concerned that he may have symptoms suggestive of renal cancer

a. List the common presenting symptoms of renal cell carcinoma
b. Describe how you would investigate this patient

Unfortunately, the results of the investigations you have ordered indicate that the patient has a left renal cell carcinoma

c. How is renal cell carcinoma staged?
d. On reviewing the patient's bloods tests, you note that the patient has a Hb of 17 g/dL. What is a possible cause of his polycythaemia?

---

AJCC TNM, American Joint Committee on Cancer, Tumor, Node and Metastases; CT, computed tomography; GP, general practitioner; Hb, haemoglobin; IV, intravenous; SCC, squamous cell carcinoma; TCC, transitional cell carcinoma

# EXPLANATION: RENAL ONCOLOGY (I)

## BENIGN KIDNEY TUMOURS

Tumours of the renal tract can occur at any site between the kidneys and the urethra. They can be divided into benign or malignant. The benign tumours can be renal papillary or metanephric adenomas which are found incidentally. Risk factors for these tumours include scarred kidneys, increasing age, polycystic kidneys and long-term haemodialysis. The other type of benign renal tract tumour is a renal oncocytoma, which is more common in 50-year-olds and males. These often present with haematuria or as a loin mass. All tumours should be considered malignant until proven otherwise.

## MALIGNANT KIDNEY TUMOURS

- **Nephroblastoma (Wilms' tumour)**: usually occurs in children under the age of 5 years. It accounts for 10 per cent of all childhood malignancies and is bilateral in 10 per cent of cases. It is associated with *WT-1* gene mutation on chromosome 11 and presents with failure to thrive, loin mass and haematuria.
- **Renal cell carcinoma** (adenocarcinoma): occurs at a mean age of 55 years and is twice as common in males:
  - clear cell carcinoma (hypernephroma, Grawitz tumour): accounts for 80 per cent of all renal cancers. It is characterized by pseudoencapsulated tumours with areas of cystic changes and calcification. At microscopy, clear cells (lipid and glycogen filled) are evident
  - chromophil cell cancer: has a better prognosis than the above. It is characterized by well-circumscribed encapsulated tumours with a friable cut surface.

Patients often present with haematuria, abdominal pain, loin mass, anorexia, paraneoplastic syndromes such as polycythaemia (erythropoeitin) **(44d)**, hypertension (renin) and hypercalcaemia (parathyroid hormone). Males can present with a left varicocele due to renal vein invasion or compression (left testicular vein drains into the left renal vein) **(44a)**. Metastasis is either due to direct spread via the renal capsule, via the lymphatics to the para-aortic nodes, or haematogenously to the liver, bone or lung (cannon ball metastases). Renal tumours can be staged using the Robson criteria (corresponding to AJCC TNM staging) **(44c)**:

- I confined to the kidney (T1 ≤7 cm; T2 >7 cm)
- II involvement of the perinephric fat but not Gerota's fascia (T3a)
- III spread into the renal vein and inferior vena cava (T3b – below diaphragm, T3c – above diaphragm)
- IV spread into adjacent or distant organs (T4).

**Pelvic tumours** arise in the uroepithelial lining and can be transitional cell carcinoma (TCC) or squamous cell carcinoma (SCC). The latter is associated with chronic irritation such as chronic stones.

Patients should be investigated with urine microscopy and cytology, blood sampling and imaging, including a chest X-ray, renal ultrasound, CT of the chest, abdomen and pelvis, echocardiogram (if staging ≥T3c) and IV urography **(44b)**.

Management options can be:

- **Palliative radiotherapy and chemotherapy**. Interleukin-2 therapy is also used for palliation
- **Surgical**: nephrectomy is the treatment of choice. Nephro-uretectomy is used for TCC. The 5-year survival following surgical therapy is approximately 98 per cent for T1 tumours and 60 per cent for T2–T3b tumours.

Answers

**42.** F T F T T
**43.** T T F F T
**44.** See explanation

### 45. Regarding bladder cancers

a. Squamous cell carcinoma is the commonest form of bladder cancer
b. Cystoscopy is used for staging
c. They are more common in women due to the higher risk of chronic urinary tract infection in women
d. Painful haematuria is classically indicative of bladder cancer until proven otherwise
e. They can present with hydronephrosis

### 46. Regarding risk factors for bladder cancer

a. Schistosomiasis is usually caused by *Schistosoma japonicum*
b. Clinical features of schistosomiasis classically occur 4–6 weeks after exposure
c. Auramine and chlorinated hydrocarbons are risk factors
d. Smoking is an important risk factor
e. Old age is a risk factor

### 47. Regarding management and presentation of bladder cancer

a. Bladder cancer involving the superficial muscle can be sufficiently managed by transurethral resection
b. In bladder cancer haematogenous spread is often an early feature and hence it presents late
c. Renal transitional cell carcinomas are best managed by nephrectomy
d. Intravesical mitomycin therapy is reserved for Tis–T2-stage bladder cancer
e. Bladder cancer lymphatic spread occurs to the inguinal nodes

### 48. Discuss the staging and prognosis of bladder cancer

SCC, squamous cell carcinoma; TCC, transitional cell carcinoma

## EXPLANATION: RENAL ONCOLOGY (II)

Bladder carcinoma is four times more prevalent in men, presenting most commonly in those over the age of 40 years. Predisposing factors include:

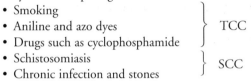

- Smoking
- Aniline and azo dyes                          } TCC
- Drugs such as cyclophosphamide
- Schistosomiasis                               } SCC
- Chronic infection and stones
- Presence of urachal remnants          Adenocarcinoma

**The commonest type of bladder cancer is TCC.** Bladder cancers are most commonly found at the trigone. They are morphologically divided into flat *in situ*, papillary, solid infiltrating and a combination of the latter two. Bladder tumours are staged as follows (48):

- Tis: carcinoma *in-situ*
- T1: limited to the lamina propria or subepithelial tissue
- T2: superficial muscle involvement
- T3: deep muscle involved, and through the bladder wall
- T4: adjacent organ involvement.

The tumour spreads either by direct extension into the pelvic viscera or by lymphatic spread to the iliac and para-aortic nodes. Haematogenous spread to the liver and lungs is a late feature.

Bladder tumours can present with painless haematuria, lower urinary tract symptoms, acute and chronic retention secondary to clot retention, or tumour-associated bladder neck obstruction. In advanced cases, chronic renal failure and hydronephrosis secondary to ureteric orifice obstruction may occur.

The investigations are similar to those for renal tumours and haematuria. However, cystoscopy and examination under anaesthesia play a vital role in investigation and management.

Management depends on the stage of the tumour. The following are possible treatment options:

- **Tis–T2**
  - trans-urethral resection of bladder tumour
  - intravesical chemotherapeutic agent, e.g. mitomycin, BCG
  - regular cystoscopic follow-up (6 months) as there is a 70 per cent chance of recurrence
- **T3–T4**
  - non-metastatic disease: radical cystectomy and reconstruction or urinary diversion, e.g. with an ileal conduit
  - metastatic disease: radiotherapy ± surgical debulking.

The prognosis is stage dependent (48):

- T1: 75 per cent 5-year survival
- T2: 50 per cent 5-year survival
- T3: 30 per cent 5-year survival
- T4: median survival of 1 year.

Answers

**45.** F T F F T
**46.** T T T T T
**47.** T F F T F
**48.** See explanation

**49. Regarding urinary tract infections**

    **a.** The most common pathogen is *Escherichia coli*
    **b.** They may be caused by parasites
    **c.** 10 per cent of women have at least one episode of UTI in their lifetime
    **d.** Asymptomatic bacteriuria in a 25-year-old female requires antibiotic treatment
    **e.** In men recurrent UTIs should be further investigated to rule out secondary causes such as obstruction

**50. Risk factors for urinary tract infection include**

    **a.** Male gender
    **b.** Pregnancy
    **c.** Diabetes mellitus
    **d.** Frequent use of antibiotics
    **e.** Vesicoureteric reflux

**51. The following are symptoms of a lower urinary tract infection**

    **a.** Haematuria
    **b.** Flank pain
    **c.** Rigors
    **d.** Dysuria
    **e.** Loin mass

**52. Acute renal infections**

    **a.** Such as pyelonephritis are associated with both acute and chronic renal failure
    **b.** Can be associated with shock
    **c.** Such as pyelonephritis usually present with lower urinary tract symptoms
    **d.** May require drainage of abscesses early
    **e.** Can result from skin infections

**53. A 45-year-old Indian immigrant presents with weight loss, urinary frequency and haematuria. Urine microscopy and culture reveals red cells, white cells but no organisms**

    **a.** How would you further investigate this patient?
    **b.** What is the most likely diagnosis?
    **c.** What are the differential diagnoses?

Ig, immunoglobulin; TB, tuberculosis; UTI, urinary tract infection

# EXPLANATION: URINARY TRACT INFECTION (I)

Urinary tract infection (UTI) is defined as the presence of a pure growth of at least **$10^5$ bacteria/mL of freshly voided urine**. The chief defence systems against a UTI are continuous urine flow (bladder washout), intermittent voiding and innate mucosal defence mechanisms (IgA and defensin secretion, urothelium phagocytic activity). Disruption of these defence mechanisms increase the risk of UTI. The major risk factors for UTI include:

- **Female sex**: it is more common in women between the ages of 1 and 60 years, because of the shorter urethra and closer proximity of the urethral opening to the anus in females. Approximately 35 per cent of women have at least one episode of UTI in their lifetime
- **Sexual intercourse**
- **Pregnancy**
- **Menopause**
- **Vaginal spermicide and diaphragm use**: there is alteration of vaginal flora
- **Diabetes mellitus**
- **Urinary tract obstruction**: including calculi, cystocele, prostatic disease, neuropathic bladder, tumours
- **Vesicoureteric reflux**
- **A foreign body** such as a urinary catheter
- **Use of immunosuppressants**
- **Renal transplantation**.

Pathogens responsible are as follows:
- **Bacteria**:
  - Gram-negative bacilli: *Escherichia coli, Klebsiella* sp., *Proteus* sp., *Pseudomonas* sp.
  - Gram-positive cocci: *Streptococcus faecalis, Staphylococcus aureus, Staphylococcus saprophyticus, Staphylococcus epidermidis*
  - *Mycobacterium tuberculosis*
- **Fungi**:
  - *Candida, Histoplasma*
- **Parasites**:
  - *Schistosoma* sp., *Echinococcus* sp.
- **Viruses**:
  - Cytomegalovirus, Adenovirus type II.

The clinical features can be divided into upper urinary tract symptoms (loin pain, fever, rigors, flank tenderness and loin mass) and lower urinary tract symptoms (dysuria, frequency, urgency, haematuria and suprapubic tenderness).

Continued on page 41

Answers
**49.** T T F F T
**50.** F T T F T
**51.** T F F T F
**52.** T T F T T
**53.** a and b – See explanation (page 41), c – The differential diagnoses are renal TB, renal cell carcinoma and bladder carcinoma

### 54. The following can be detected by urine dipstick

    **a.** Bence Jones protein
    **b.** Microalbuminuria
    **c.** Leucocytes
    **d.** Red cell casts
    **e.** White blood cells

### 55. The following meet the criteria for bacteriuria

    **a.** $\geq 10^5$ coliform organisms/mL urine plus pyuria in a 25-year-old female with dysuria
    **b.** Any growth of organisms in urine obtained by suprapubic aspiration in an 18-year-old female with dysuria
    **c.** $\geq 10^2$ pathogenic organisms/mL urine in a 50-year-old male
    **d.** $\geq 10^5$ pathogenic organisms/mL urine on two occasions in an asymptomatic adult
    **e.** $\geq 10^2$ pathogenic organisms/mL urine, with urgency, in a 27-year-old woman

### 56. Consider management of urinary tract infection

    **a.** In all cases it requires a renal ultrasound
    **b.** Patients should be advised about fluid intake and perineal hygiene
    **c.** Pyelonephritis is best treated with IV penicillin
    **d.** Renal TB requires quadruple therapy for 12 months to ensure eradication
    **e.** For a simple UTI, a 3-day course of antibiotics is often sufficient

### 57. In recurrent urinary tract infections, describe the differences between reinfection and relapse

---

AFB, acid-fast bacilli; ESRF, end-stage renal failure; IV, intravenous; UTI, urinary tract infection; TB, tuberculosis

## EXPLANATION: URINARY TRACT INFECTION (I)  Cont'd from page 39

### UTI CLINICAL SYNDROMES

- **Asymptomatic bacteriuria**: found in 5 per cent of 15-year-olds. It does not require treatment except in pregnancy (associated with increased risk of pre-term labour), in the young with vesicoureteric reflux and prior to urological procedures.
- **Sterile pyuria**: the presence of raised white cells in urine (>20 cells/mm$^3$) without bacteriuria can be due to incomplete antibiotic treatment, atypical organisms, vaginal leucocyte contamination, chronic interstitial nephritis, or the presence of a tumour or stones.
- **Acute urethral syndrome**: this syndrome is common in women. It presents with lower urinary tract symptoms, but there is no bacteriuria.
- **Acute cystitis**: the patient presents with lower urinary tract symptoms and signs. The patient is classically not systemically unwell. Recurrence of cystitis can be due to inadequate treatment (relapse – bacteriuria with the same organism within 7 days of completing antibiotic treatment) or re-infection (with an identical or different organism after the absence of bacteriuria for at least 14 days following treatment).
- **Acute renal infections**: usually from an ascending infection, they can also arise from haematogenous spread. Urine-borne infection has a characteristic wedge-shaped inflammation from the calices to the cortex, while haematogenous infection leads to diffuse inflammation. If associated with an obstruction, there is rapid renal parenchyma destruction.
  - acute pyelonephritis – renal parenchymal inflammation
  - renal carbuncle – abscess within the renal parenchyma is usually confined to the cortex. More commonly it is due to haematogenous spread of organisms, e.g. *Staphylococcus aureus* from a skin infection. It is seen in diabetics and IV drug users
  - pyonephrosis – rapid renal tissue destruction as a result of an infection associated with obstruction
  - perinephric abscess – can result from any of the above, and is initially confined by Gerota's fascia. It can rupture and reach the psoas muscle, bowel, pleura or skin in Petit's lumbar triangle. The patient often has scoliosis with concavity towards the affected side.

  The patient presents with upper urinary tract symptoms and signs. If left untreated it can progress to septic shock.
- **Chronic pyelonephritis**: characterized by a combination of renal scarring and urinary infection. It usually follows vesicoureteric reflux and infection in childhood. It can also occur as a result of repeated episodes of acute pyelonephritis. It accounts for 30 per cent of ESRF cases in childhood.
- **Renal TB (53b)**: a classical cause of sterile pyuria, usually as a result of spread from a pulmonary focus. Heaf or Mantoux tests are usually positive in these patients. It is usually diagnosed by identification of acid-fast bacilli (AFB) in three early-morning urine samples **(53a)**. Patients are prone to ureteric strictures following renal TB.

Answers
**54.** F F T F T
**55.** T T F T F
**56.** F T F F T
**57.** See explanation (page 42)

# EXPLANATION: URINARY TRACT INFECTION (II)

**Investigations** should be tailored to the patient's needs. Women with recurrent UTIs, children and men need rigorous investigations as they are more likely to have an underlying cause.

- Urinary sampling: midstream urine (MSU), catheter specimen, suprapubic needle aspiration and, rarely, prostatic massage:
  - general appearance – hazy urine
  - urine dipstick – often positive for blood, protein, nitrites and leucocytes
  - urine MC&S: characterized by $>10^3$ organisms/mL urine (men) or $>10^5$ organisms/mL urine (women). If a suprapubic specimen is obtained, any growth is significant
  - early-morning urine samples for AFB
- Blood sampling: full blood count (raised WCC), renal function, CRP, blood cultures
- Imaging: KUB X-ray, renal ultrasound, IV urogram, micturating cystogram, DMSA scan.

## MANAGEMENT

Collection of urine for MC&S before treatment is desirable. However, in primary care in a woman with uncomplicated cystitis, a positive dipstick test for nitrite and leucocyte esterase is considered sufficient. Treatment is generally empirical while the result of urine culture is pending. Trimethoprim (200 mg twice daily) is a commonly used first-line treatment, effective against approximately 70 per cent of urinary pathogens. Nitrofurantoin (50 mg three times daily) or an oral cephalosporin are also commonly prescribed. Uncomplicated cystitis may be managed with just a 3-day course of antibiotics. However, treatment may be later modified depending on clinical response, and the results of urine culture and sensitivity. With resistant organisms, antibiotics such as ciprofloxacin may be necessary. Amoxicillin is now rarely used even in the community, with many urinary pathogens now resistant.

In women with recurrent infections, general measures such as high oral fluid intake, regular bladder empty-ing, double micturition, voiding pre- and post-sexual intercourse and good personal hygiene should be recommended. Avoidance of chemicals in bathwater, such as bubble bath, and treatment of constipation (which may lead to urinary retention) are also helpful.

When managing recurrent infections it is important to differentiate between **relapse** and **reinfection (57)**. Approximately 80 per cent of recurrent UTIs are reinfections, occurring more than 14 days after resolution of the initial infection. Importantly, this is not due to failure of eradication of the original infection, but rather the result of reinvasion of a susceptible urinary tract. The pathogen is often different from the organism suc-cessfully treated in the previous infection. Relapse is defined as the recurrence of bacteriuria with the same organisms within 7 days of completion of antimicrobial treatment. Relapses signify that the original pathogen was never eradicated, suggesting the presence of underlying factors such as scarred kidneys or stones.

Acute pyelonephritis requires hospital admission and is best treated with intravenous antibiotics such as cefuroxime or a quinolone (ciprofloxacin) to prevent complications. Renal TB requires triple therapy (rifampicin, isoniazid and pyrazinamide) for 9 months. Collections if present need to be drained.

---

AFB, acid-fast bacilli; CRP, C-reactive protein; DMSA, dimercaptosuccinic acid; FBC, full blood count; IV, intravenous; KUB, kidneys, ureters and bladder; MC&S, microscopy, culture and sensitivity; MSU, midstream urine; TB, tuberculosis; UTI, urinary tract infection; WCC, white cell count

# HEPATOBILIARY MEDICINE

# SECTION 2

# HEPATOBILIARY MEDICINE

## 1. Regarding bilirubin metabolism

a. 85 per cent of bilirubin is a result of haemoglobin degradation
b. The kidney excretes unconjugated bilirubin
c. Conjugated bilirubin is absorbed from the terminal ileum
d. Conjugation occurs in the intrahepatic bile ducts
e. Bilirubin is excreted in faeces as urobilinogen

## 2. Regarding jaundice

a. The presence of a palpable gall bladder with painless jaundice suggests a diagnosis of hepatocellular carcinoma
b. Sepsis is a cause of jaundice
c. A markedly raised alkaline phosphatase compared to other liver enzymes suggests an obstructive jaundice
d. Urobilinogen in urine is not detectable normally
e. A high urobilinogen in urine is a marker of hepatocellular dysfunction

---

ATP, adenosine triphosphate; TB, tuberculosis; UDP, uridine diphosphate; UGT, UDP glucuronyl transferase

## EXPLANATION: JAUNDICE

Jaundice is defined as a yellow discoloration of the skin, sclera and mucous membranes as a result of elevated bilirubin concentrations (clinically evident when bilirubin exceeds 35–40 µmol/L). **See Appendix, page 152 for bilirubin metabolism.**

The causes of jaundice can be classified under three main categories. They are pre-hepatic, hepatic and post-hepatic jaundice.

### PRE-HEPATIC JAUNDICE

- **Increased bilirubin production** occurs when there is increased breakdown of red blood cells, possibly due to haemolytic anaemia (sickle cell disease, malaria and drug-induced), ineffective erythropoesis, blood transfusion and re-absorption of haematoma. Another cause of pre-hepatic jaundice is a **reduced bilirubin uptake**, often secondary to drugs, such as rifampicin, which compete with bilirubin for protein binding or receptor uptake.

### HEPATIC/HEPATOCELLULAR JAUNDICE

- Unconjugated hyperbilirubinaemia:
  - **Gilbert's syndrome**: a benign autosomal recessive condition that affects about 5 per cent of the population. It is characterized by mild and intermittent jaundice following intercurrent infection or fasting. In most patients, there is a defect in the gene encoding UGT. It does not require any treatment
  - **Crigler–Najjar syndrome**: type 1 is a rare autosomal recessive condition resulting in an absence of UGT. It has a high mortality within the first year of life due to kernicterus (deposition of bilirubin in basal ganglia). Type 2 is an autosomal dominant condition with a reduced level of UGT.
- Conjugated hyperbilirubinaemia:
  - **Dubin–Johnson syndrome**: an autosomal recessive condition associated with defective ATP-dependent cannalicular transport of bile. It usually presents during pregnancy or after use of the oral contraceptive pill. The prognosis is excellent
  - **infections**: viral and bacterial hepatitis, TB
  - **hepatotoxins**: such as alcohol, paracetamol, co-amoxiclav and aflatoxins
  - **ischaemia**: due to hypotension or occlusive vascular disease (Budd–Chiari syndrome)
  - **metabolic disorders**: include Wilson's disease, haemochromatosis and $\alpha_1$-antitrypsin deficiency
  - **infiltrative disorders**: primary and metastatic tumours, sarcoidosis and amyloidosis.

Continued on page 47

Answers
1. T F T F F
2. F T T F T

3. For the following scenarios choose the most appropriate diagnosis. Each option may be used once only

**Options**

A. Hepatitis A
B. Ascending cholangitis
C. Crigler–Najjar syndrome
D. Primary biliary cirrhosis
E. Pancreatic cancer

F. Malaria
G. Gilbert's syndrome
H. Hepatocellular carcinoma
I. Hepatitis C
J. Primary sclerosing cholangitis

1. A 56-year-old smoker presents with a 3-month history of weight loss and painless jaundice. She has noticed pale stool and dark urine
2. A 50-year-old woman presents with jaundice. She noticed that over the last 3 months she has had pruritus and right upper quadrant pain. On examination she has xanthelasma and hepatosplenomegaly
3. A 52-year-old presents with jaundice following reduced oral intake during an upper respiratory tract infection. He is otherwise well and the jaundice is self-limiting
4. A 58-year-old presents with nausea, vomiting, right upper quadrant pain and jaundice. His wife has also had similar symptoms over the same time period
5. A 40-year-old presents with rigors, nausea, vomiting and jaundice following a holiday in Nigeria

4. You are asked to see a deeply jaundiced 73-year-old woman. Her blood results demonstrate a bilirubin of 445 µmol/L, alkaline phosphatase of 798 iu/L, and aspartate transaminase of 73 iu/L. She has lost 6 kg in the past 8 months

a. Is this likely to be obstructive or hepatocellular jaundice?
b. What questions could you ask to help determine the cause of the jaundice?
c. How would you further investigate this patient?
d. The patient is complaining bitterly of continuous itching. How could you manage this distressing symptom?

AFP, α-fetoprotein; ALP, alkaline phosphatase; CT, computed tomography; ERCP, endoscopic retrograde cholangiopancreatography; FBC, full blood count; GGT, γ-glutamyl transferase; MRCP, magnetic resonance cholangiopancreatography; PTC, percutaneous transhepatic cholangiography; UDP, uridine diphosphate

# EXPLANATION: JAUNDICE Cont'd from page 45

## POST-HEPATIC/OBSTRUCTIVE JAUNDICE

- Extraluminal obstruction: pancreas head carcinoma, pancreatitis, hilar lymphadenopathy and liver metastases.
- Intramural obstruction: sclerosing cholangitis, cholangiocarcinoma, Mirrizi's syndrome and inflammatory strictures.
- Intraluminal obstruction: gallstones, schistosomiasis, papilloma and tumour thrombus.

The history can help elicit the cause of jaundice **(4b)**. It is pertinent to ask about occupational exposure, foreign travel, associated symptoms, drug history and alcohol intake.

On examination, excoriations, bruises, tattoos and needle tracks may be visible. Stigmata of chronic liver disease such as leuconychia, clubbing, Dupuytren's contracture, spider naevi, testicular atrophy and parotid enlargement may be present. It is important to consider **Courvoisier's law** when palpating the abdomen. It states that painless jaundice in the presence of a palpable gall bladder is unlikely to be due to gallstones.

Important investigations in a jaundiced patient include **(4c)**:
- Blood analysis: FBC and blood film, liver profile (disproportionally high ALP suggests obstructive jaundice while high transaminases and GGT suggest hepatocellular jaundice **(4a)**), coagulation profile, renal profile, hepatitis screen and autoimmune profile. It may be necessary to perform other tests such as blood ferritin, caeruloplasmin, tumour markers e.g. CA 19-9, AFP
- Imaging studies: ultrasound, CT scan, endoscopic retrograde cholangiopancreatography (ERCP, which can be diagnostic and therapeutic), percutaneous transhepatic cholangiography (PTC), magnetic resonance cholangiopancreatography (MRCP).

Treat the underlying condition. Pruritus can be managed by antihistamines, cholestyramine, rifampicin or ursodeoxycholic acid **(4d)**.

---

## Answers
**3.** 1 – E, 2 – D, 3 – G, 4 – A, 5 – F
**4.** See explanation

## 5. Regarding acute liver failure

**a.** Paracetamol overdose is the commonest cause in the UK
**b.** The presence of Babinski's sign suggests a grade IV encephalopathy
**c.** Liver transplantation is indicated for paracetamol poisoning with a blood bilirubin concentration >300 $\mu$mol/L
**d.** Drug hypersensitivity is a common complication
**e.** Candidaemia is a known complication

ALF, acute liver failure

## EXPLANATION: LIVER FAILURE (I)

Hepatic failure is defined as a state in which the liver is unable to adequately perform its many functions, characterized by abnormalities in protein synthesis, lipid and carbohydrate metabolism, bile secretion and metabolism, as well as nitrogen excretion.

Liver failure can be classified into two categories, acute and chronic.

**Acute liver failure** (ALF) is often characterized by encephalopathy; the patient becomes unwell within 24–48 h. Fulminant liver failure is a subtype where there is a progression from normal liver function to liver failure within 8 weeks. Subacute liver failure is defined as the presence of liver disease for up to 26 weeks prior to the development of hepatic encephalopathy.

In the UK, **paracetamol overdose** is the commonest cause of ALF, but worldwide, **viral hepatitis** accounts for the majority of cases. Other causes are summarized below:
- **Drugs**:
  - paracetamol overdose
  - antituberculous drugs
  - halothane
- **Infection**:
  - hepatitis A, B, E
  - herpes simplex virus
- **Vascular**:
  - ischaemia
  - Budd–Chiari syndrome: an uncommon condition characterized by hepatic venous drainage obstruction (thrombotic or non-thrombotic)
- **Toxins**:
  - carbon tetrachloride
  - amanita phalloides
- **Others**:
  - acute fatty liver of pregnancy
  - Wilson's disease (disorder of copper metabolism)
  - lymphoma.

Continued on page 51

Answer

**5.** T F F F F

### 6. Regarding the grading of encephalopathy

a. Encephalopathy is graded I–V
b. Sleep pattern reversal and apraxia occur in grade I encephalopathy
c. The presence of Babinski's sign suggests a grade IV encephalopathy
d. Hyporeflexia is a sign of grade III encephalopathy
e. Grade IV encephalopathy is associated with coma

### 7. A 35-year-old male presents to the emergency department in acute liver failure following a paracetamol overdose. He is at risk of the following complications

a. Hyperglycaemia
b. Candidaemia
c. Renal failure
d. GI haemorrhage
e. Pulmonary oedema

### 8. For the following scenarios choose the most appropriate diagnosis. Each option may be used once only

**Options**

A. Carcinoid syndrome
B. Portal vein thrombosis
C. Constrictive pericarditis
D. Tuberculosis
E. Meig's syndrome
F. Pseudomyxoma peritonei
G. Right-sided heart failure
H. Ectopic pregnancy
I. Secondary to metastatic deposits
J. Budd–Chiari syndrome

1. A 30-year-old woman who has recently started on the oral contraceptive pill develops right upper quadrant pain and a distended abdomen. On examination she has hepatomegaly and shifting dullness on percussion, with a fluid thrill
2. A 64-year-old man presents with longstanding fatigue and shortness of breath. On examination he has a small volume pulse, raised jugular venous pressure and soft heart sounds. He also has ascites and peripheral oedema
3. A 29-year-old woman with sudden-onset right iliac fossa pain and a positive pregnancy test is found to have haemorrhagic intraperitoneal fluid at laparoscopy
4. A 75-year-old patient with a past medical history of a right hemicolectomy for a caecal mass now presents with weight loss and ascites
5. A 26-year-old man with right iliac fossa pain is explored at laparotomy, which demonstrated a viscous mucinoid collection of intraperitoneal fluid and an appendiceal mass

---

CT, computed tomography; GCS, Glasgow Coma Scale; GI, gastrointestinal; HDU, high-dependency unit; ITU, intensive therapy unit; IV, intravenous

## EXPLANATION: LIVER FAILURE (I) Cont'd from page 49

The patient often presents with:
- Jaundice
- Encephalopathy which is graded as follows:
  - grade I: altered mood, sleep pattern reversal, apraxia
  - grade II: drowsiness, confusion, asterixis, ataxia, hyporeflexia
  - grade III: stupor, Babinski's sign, hyper-reflexia
  - grade IV: coma, decerebration
- Hypoglycaemia
- Haemorrhage (failure to synthesize clotting factors)
- Infections (bacterial and fungal)
- Renal failure (hepatorenal syndrome).

The investigations required are as with any patient with jaundice. Furthermore, an arterial blood gas sample must be taken with blood, urine and, if present, ascitic fluid cultures to exclude infection. A liver ultrasound and CT of the abdomen are helpful.

Patients may require ITU or HDU care. A nasogastric tube may be inserted to minimize aspiration, and endotracheal intubation should be considered if the GCS is low (<7–8). Proton pump inhibitors are administered IV to reduce the risk of a GI bleed. Coagulopathy is managed with IV vitamin K. Fresh-frozen plasma is only used in the presence of active bleeding, as the prothrombin time is an important predictor of outcome. Platelet concentrates are used if the platelet count is $<50 \times 10^9/L$ and there is active bleeding.

There is no good clinical evidence supporting protein restriction in patients with acute hepatic encephalopathy. Lactulose is given either orally or by enema to minimize nitrogenous substance absorption via the GI tract. Hepatorenal syndrome is managed with adequate intravascular filling with colloids such as albumin; vasopressin analogues are also used. Dialysis is reserved for particular indications such as severe metabolic acidosis, hyperkalaemia and pulmonary oedema.

The King's College Hospital criteria are used to identify situations where liver transplantation may be of benefit:

| Paracetamol poisoning | Other scenarios |
|---|---|
| • pH <7.3 24 h after ingestion<br>OR the combination of:<br>  • Prothrombin time >100 s<br>  • Creatinine >300 µmol/L<br>  • ≥ Grade III encephalopathy | • Prothrombin time >100 s<br>OR ≥3 of the following:<br>  • Drug or non-viral hepatitis<br>  • Age <10 years or >40 years<br>  • Jaundice present for >7 days prior to encephalopathy<br>  • Blood bilirubin >300 µmol/L<br>  • Prothrombin time >50 s |

## 9. Regarding chronic liver failure

**a.** In Wilson's disease the presence of excess copper in the liver histology is diagnostic
**b.** Wilson's disease characteristically has a raised blood caeruloplasmin level
**c.** Haemochromatosis is more common in females
**d.** Hepatitis A is a known cause
**e.** Amiodarone is a cause

## 10. Regarding haemochromatosis

**a.** It is an autosomal dominant condition
**b.** It is more common in males
**c.** It may present with diabetes
**d.** The patient may have bronzed skin
**e.** Regular venesection is a possible treatment

---

AAT, $\alpha_1$-antitrypsin; CLF, chronic liver failure; CT, computed tomography; GI, gastrointestinal; MRI, magnetic resonance imaging; SLE, systemic lupus erythematosus; TIPS, transjugular intrahepatic portosystemic shunt

## EXPLANATION: LIVER FAILURE (II)

**Chronic liver failure (CLF)/cirrhosis** is described as irreversible liver damage resulting from diffuse fibrosis and nodular regeneration. The causes of CLF are summarized below:
• Alcohol
• Infection: viral hepatitis B, C and D, schistosomiasis
• Metabolic:
  • **primary biliary cirrhosis**
  • **autoimmune hepatitis**
  • **haemochromatosis**: an autosomal recessive condition (point mutation in the *HFE* gene) that results in increased iron absorption from the GI tract and deposition in various organs. The male:female ratio is 10:1. The condition classically presents in a middle-aged man with bronzed skin pigmentation, diabetes, cardiac failure and hepatomegaly. Patients have a raised blood iron, ferritin and transferrin saturation level. Treatment options include regular venesection, iron-chelating agents (desferrioxamine) and liver transplantation
  • **Wilson's disease**: a rare autosomal recessive disorder of copper metabolism (copper-transporting ATPase mutation) characterized by accumulation of copper in the major organs. Adults present with neurological symptoms such as tremor, dysarthria, Parkinsonian symptoms and dementia. Classically Kayser–Fleischer rings due to copper deposition in Descemet's membrane may be present. Blood copper and caeruloplasmin levels are low, with an elevated urinary copper level. A liver biopsy demonstrates high hepatic copper levels. This condition is managed with the use of the chelating agents D-penicillamine and trientine dihydrochloride. Liver transplantation is reserved for fulminant forms
  • **$\alpha_1$-antitrypsin (AAT) deficiency**: this is an autosomal dominant condition that primarily manifests as panacinar emphysema. AAT is normally produced by hepatocytes and protects the alveoli against protease destruction. Symptoms of emphysema develop in the fourth (smokers) or fifth (non-smokers) decade. The genotype ZZ is responsible for most cases (normal genotype is MM). A minority of patients (about 10 per cent) develop hepatic cirrhosis. Treatment involves cessation of smoking, pulmonary rehabilitation, intravenous augmentation therapy with pooled human AAT and lung transplantation
• Prolonged cholestasis
• Hepatic venous outflow obstruction
  • **Budd–Chiari syndrome**: this syndrome results due to thrombotic or non-thrombotic occlusion of the hepatic veins. The causes include: polycythaemia vera, paroxysmal nocturnal haemoglobinuria, thrombotic disorders, pregnancy, oral contraceptive pill use, malignancy, SLE, hepatocellular carcinoma, venous webs and radiotherapy. It classically presents with a triad of abdominal pain, ascites (high protein content) and hepatomegaly. Ultrasound, CT or MRI will demonstrate the occlusion. The congested liver is decompressed with a transjugular intrahepatic portosystemic shunt (TIPS) or side-to-side portocaval or splenorenal anastomosis. Liver transplantation is considered for the chronic cases. Most patients also receive anticoagulation
  • **constrictive pericarditis**
  • **heart failure**
• Drugs such as amiodarone and methotrexate.

Continued on page 55

Answers
**9.** F F F F T
**10.** F T T T T

## 11. Regarding the Child–Pugh criteria

a. There are four stages
b. They are of value in determining prognosis
c. Nutrition is scored
d. The patient's serum ALP is assessed
e. The patient's serum albumin is assessed

## 12. For the following scenarios, choose the most appropriate blood test

**Options**

A. Serum caeruloplasmin
B. Paracetamol level
C. α-fetoprotein
D. $\alpha_1$-antitrypsin
E. Hepatitis serology
F. Antimitochondrial antibody
G. Serum glucose
H. Thrombophilia screen
I. Serum ferritin
J. Antinuclear, liver/kidney microsomal and smooth muscle antibody

1. A 45-year-old newly diagnosed patient with diabetes presents with signs of pulmonary oedema, a swollen left knee and a bronzed tinge to his skin
2. A 53-year-old female complains of worsening shortness of breath, and jaundice. She has smoked since the age of 15 years. Her family history reveals that her father, who never smoked, died of 'longstanding breathing difficulties' in his 60s
3. A 17-year-old female presents to her GP with tremor, dysarthria and dyskinesia. On examination, the patient has a greenish pigment in the peripheral cornea
4. A 51-year-old female complains of pruritus. On examination, she has xanthelasma and hepatomegaly, but is not jaundiced
5. A 35-year-old female with known hyperthyroidism and diabetes presents with jaundice and ascites. She drinks three glasses of wine a week

AFP, α-fetoprotein; ALF, acute liver failure; ALP, alkaline phosphatase; GP, general practitioner

## EXPLANATION: LIVER FAILURE (II) Cont'd from page 53

The investigation and management of CLF is similar to that of ALF. Patients should be followed up regularly with imaging and testing of AFP levels due to the high risk of hepatocellular carcinoma.

Good prognostic indicators in cirrhosis are summarized by the Child–Pugh criteria:

|  | Stage | | |
| --- | --- | --- | --- |
|  | A | B | C |
| Blood bilirubin (μmol/L) | <34.2 | 34.2–51.3 | >51.3 |
| Blood albumin (g/L) | >35 | 30–35 | <30 |
| Ascites | None | Easily controlled | Poorly controlled |
| Neurological disorder | None | Minimal | Comatosed |
| Nutrition | Excellent | Good | Poor |

The differential diagnosis of ascites can be categorized according to fluid type: **haemorrhagic fluid** (malignancy, trauma, pancreatitis and ectopic pregnancy), **chylous fluid** (malignancy and cirrhosis) and **straw-coloured fluid** (malignancy, cirrhosis, heart failure, constrictive pericarditis, hypoproteinaemia states e.g. protein-losing enteropathy and nephrotic syndrome, infection, pancreatitis and Meig's syndrome).

Answers
**11.** F T T F T
**12.** 1 – I, 2 – D, 3 – A, 4 – F, 5 – J

### 13. Regarding viral hepatitis

a. 50 per cent of those infected with hepatitis B in adulthood become chronic carriers
b. Hepatitis A infection is associated with shellfish intake
c. Hepatitis B is an RNA virus
d. The presence of the e antigen indicates increased infectivity
e. Lamivudine is a therapeutic option for hepatitis C

### 14. The following are well-known causes of chronic hepatitis

a. Alcohol
b. Hepatitis C
c. Granulomatous disease
d. $\alpha_1$-antitrypsin deficiency
e. Hepatitis E

### 15. Regarding hepatitis B

a. It is spread via the oro-faecal route
b. It may be associated with arthralgia
c. The presence of HBeAg implies high infectivity
d. A carrier status has been described following infection
e. Hepatocellular carcinoma is a possible complication

DNA, deoxyribonucleic acid; HB, hepatitis B; IV, intravenous; RNA, ribonucleic acid

## EXPLANATION: VIRAL HEPATITIS

Acute **viral hepatitis** presents with a short-lived acute illness that is rarely fatal, but pregnant and immuno-compromised patients can be debilitated. However, some types of hepatitis virus result in chronic disease. There are six confirmed types of hepatitis virus:

1. **Hepatitis A (RNA virus)**: this virus has an incubation period of 2–8 weeks and is transmitted via the oro-faecal route. Community outbreaks due to contaminated water or food, usually shellfish, may also occur. There are no cases of chronic infection. Patients present with symptoms such as malaise, anorexia, nausea, vomiting, pruritus and a dull right upper quadrant abdominal pain. Clinical signs include jaundice and hepatomegaly. Preventative vaccination is available. Treatment involves supportive care. There is no role for antivirals or steroid therapy

2. **Hepatitis B (DNA virus)**: the incubation period is 2–4 months. The virus is transmitted via blood-borne or sexual contact. Seventy-five per cent of patients have non-specific symptoms or may remain asymptomatic; 5 per cent of acute infections progress to chronic infection. An effective vaccine is available. In the acute setting therapy is supportive. **Interferon-α** has been used for chronic cases, with approximately 25 per cent of patients becoming carrier free. Monotherapy with the reverse transcription inhibitor **lamivudine** reduces viral load and serum alanine transaminase in most patients, with the nucleotide ana-logue **adefovir** reserved for those who develop lamivudine resistance.

3. **Hepatitis C (RNA virus)**: this virus has an incubation period of 2–6 weeks and has similar modes of transmission as hepatitis B. Only 30 per cent of patients develop symptomatic acute infection; 80 per cent of acute infections result in chronic infection. There is no vaccine available at present. Treatment with **interferon-α** effectively eradicates the virus in 10 per cent of cases. There are better response rates with **ribavirin** combination therapy

4. **Hepatitis D (RNA virus)**: this is a defective RNA virus that requires co-infection with hepatitis B for complete viral assembly and secretion, so it is unable to cause infection solely. It usually presents as co-infection or super-infection in IV drug users. There is a high risk of acute hepatic failure and cirrhosis. No vaccine is available

5. **Hepatitis E (RNA virus)**: this virus is primarily found in Southeast Asia. It is transmitted through the oro-faecal route. Fulminant hepatitis can occur, particularly in women in the third trimester of pregnancy. There is no effective vaccine or chronic infection

6. **Hepatitis G (RNA virus)**: this virus can be spread by transfusion of contaminated blood, in a similar way to hepatitis B and C. Most evidence suggests that hepatitis G virus is not a cause of acute hepatitis or chronic liver disease.

Continued on page 59

Answers

**13.** F T F T F
**14.** T T T T F
**15.** F T T T T

16. For the following statements, choose the most appropriate answer. Each option may be used once only

## Options

**A.** Hepatitis A

**B.** Hepatitis B

**C.** Hepatitis C

**D.** Hepatitis D

**E.** Hepatitis E

**F.** Hepatitis G

1. A defective RNA virus that is unable to cause infection in the absence of hepatitis B
2. Outbreaks may occur as a result of contaminated shellfish. A preventative vaccine is available
3. Infection is of particular concern in pregnant women
4. A DNA virus
5. A blood-borne virus for which there is no effective vaccine

Ag, antigen; ALP, alkaline phosphatase; ALT, alanine transaminase; AST, aspartate transaminase; DNA, deoxyribonucleic acid; HB, hepatitis B; Ig, immunoglobulin; RNA, ribonucleic acid

## EXPLANATION: VIRAL HEPATITIS Cont'd from page 57

The laboratory studies in viral hepatitis often show a marked rise in enzymes released by hepatocyte lysis including aspartate and alanine transaminase enzymes (AST and ALT, respectively). There are no or minimal rises in alkaline phosphatase (ALP) levels.

Serological tests are often difficult to interpret in viral hepatitis associated with chronic infection. The table below summarizes the possible serology results and the relevance for hepatitis B (HB):

| HBsAg | HBeAg | Anti-HBe | Anti-HBc IgM | IgG | Anti-HBs | Interpretation |
|-------|-------|----------|--------------|-----|----------|----------------|
| + | + | − | + | + | − | Acute or carrier state |
| + | +/− | +/− | +/− | + | − | Persistent carrier state |
| − | − | − | − | + | + | Distant infection |
| − | − | − | − | − | + | Immunization without infection |

Chronic hepatitis has a varied course. It can progress to the development of cirrhosis and portal hypertension. Hepatocellular carcinoma develops in up to 25 per cent of chronic hepatitis B patients, and is often multifocal in these cases. Chronic hepatitis C related to blood transfusions has an increased incidence of cirrhosis.

Answer

**16.** 1 – D, 2 – A, 3 – E, 4 – B, 5 – C

## 17. Regarding autoimmune hepatitis

a. It is a common cause of hepatitis
b. There is an association with other autoimmune disorders
c. Type 1 is associated with antinuclear antibodies
d. Type 2 is more common in children
e. Immunosuppressive therapy may be used if there is active inflammation

## 18. Regarding primary biliary cirrhosis

a. It is much more common in females
b. It usually presents in those >60 years old
c. It is associated with breast cancer
d. Patients usually have antimitochondrial antibodies
e. It often presents with pruritus

## 19. Regarding primary sclerosing cholangitis

a. It is twice as common in males
b. 5 per cent of patients with primary sclerosing cholangitis have ulcerative colitis
c. Retroperitoneal fibrosis is a complication
d. ERCP shows biliary tree stricturing and beading
e. Immunosuppressants are usually effective

## 20. A 47-year-old female is newly diagnosed with primary biliary cirrhosis

a. How might she have presented?
b. What conditions is primary biliary cirrhosis commonly associated with?
c. Discuss the available management options. What is this patient's prognosis?

---

AMA, antimitochondrial antibody; ANA, antinuclear antibody; ANCA, antineutrophil cytoplasmic antibody; ERCP, endoscopic retrograde cholangiopancreatography; HLA, human leucocyte antigen; Ig, immunoglobulin; PBC, primary biliary cirrhosis; PSC, primary sclerosing cholangitis

## EXPLANATION: AUTOIMMUNE LIVER DISEASE

**Autoimmune hepatitis** is a rare inflammatory liver disease of unknown origin associated with autoimmune disorders, the presence of autoantibodies and hyperglobulinaemia. It is more common in young females who often have a personal or family history of other autoimmune disorders. There are two main types:
- Type 1: can affect all age groups and is associated with antinuclear antibodies (ANA) and/or smooth muscle antibodies. Recent reclassification of autoimmune hepatitis has also included patients with anti-soluble liver-pancreas antibodies (formerly type 3 autoimmune hepatitis) into this subgroup
- Type 2: more common in children, this is associated with anti-liver-kidney microsomal antibodies. This subtype is especially associated with type 1 diabetes mellitus, autoimmune thyroiditis and vitiligo.

Both subtypes may present with an acute or chronic hepatitis picture. The management options for autoimmune hepatitis include immunosuppressive therapy with corticosteroid ± azathioprine in patients with active inflammation. Approximately 15 per cent of patients have no relapse after 2 years of immunosuppression. In cases of end-stage hepatitis and cirrhosis, liver transplantation is the treatment of choice.

**Primary biliary cirrhosis (PBC)** is a granulomatous inflammatory condition that affects interlobular bile ducts leading to fibrosis and cirrhosis. The condition usually presents in females (M:F = 1:9) in the 40–60 years age range. There is a **strong association with other autoimmune conditions** such as Sicca syndrome (characterized by dry mouth and eyes), rheumatoid arthritis and autoimmune thyroid disease, as well as breast cancer, hepatocellular carcinoma and pancreatic insufficiency **(20b)**. Patients with the condition usually have antimitochondrial antibodies (AMA, anti-M2). PBC may be asymptomatic or present insidiously with **(20a)**: pruritis without jaundice, lethargy and fatigue, jaundice (occurs 6–48 months later), chronic right upper quadrant pain, hepatosplenomegaly, xanthelasma or xanthomata.

The management options include **(20c)**:
- Nutrition: fat-soluble vitamins (A, D, E and K) as well as calcium supplements
- Pruritus management with antihistamines, cholestyramine, ursodeoxycholic acid. The latter is especially useful in PBC as it also reduces HLA class I expression on bile ducts, reducing Tc cell attack
- Liver transplantation: offers the best prognosis.

Asymptomatic patients have a life expectancy of approximately 10 years, while symptomatic or jaundiced patients have a poor survival prospect of less than 2 years.

**Primary sclerosing cholangitis (PSC)** is a cholestatic liver disease of unknown cause resulting in diffuse biliary inflammation, fibrosis and strictures. The condition is more common in men (M:F = 2:1) usually between the ages of 25 and 45 years. There is a 75 per cent association with ulcerative colitis, and the prevalence of PSC in patients with ulcerative colitis is about 5 per cent. There is a strong genetic predisposition attributable to HLA haplotype A1 B8 DR3. Patients often present with weight loss, malaise, right upper quadrant pain, pruritus and intermittent jaundice. PSC may be complicated by bacterial cholangitis, retroperitoneal fibrosis, cholangiocarcinoma (in 10–30 per cent) and colorectal cancer. Most PSC patients have raised IgM levels. About 70 per cent of cases are ANCA positive. ERCP is diagnostic, revealing generalized beading and stricturing of the biliary tree. The management options are: cholestyramine or ursodeoxycholic acid for pruritus, endoscopic biliary dilatation and stent insertion, fat-soluble vitamins (A, D, E and K), liver transplantation. Symptomatic patients have a mean survival without transplantation of 12–20 years.

Answers
**17.** F T T T T
**18.** T F T T T
**19.** T F T T F
**20.** See explanation

### 21. Regarding assessment of acute pancreatitis severity

a. The modified Glasgow criteria are reserved for those with alcohol-induced pancreatitis
b. Amylase is a determining factor of severity in the Ranson's criteria
c. Sex is a determinant of severity
d. In severe cases mortality can be as high as 20 per cent
e. Creatinine is a determining factor of severity in the Ranson's criteria

### 22. Causes of acute pancreatitis include

a. ERCP
b. Hypocalcaemia
c. Thiazide diuretics

d. Hyperlipidaemia
e. Diazepam poisoning

### 23. You are the surgical F1 doctor on-call at the weekend. You are asked to review a 70-year-old male patient with a history of alcohol abuse who was admitted 2 days ago with acute pancreatitis

**Admission blood results:**

| | |
|---|---|
| WCC | $20 \times 10^9$/L |
| Hb | 13 g/dL |
| Haematocrit | 0.54 |
| Blood glucose | 7 mmol/L |
| LDH | 478 IU/L |
| AST | 712 IU/L |
| Bilirubin | 78 $\mu$mol/L |
| Creatinine | 102 $\mu$mol/L |
| Urea | 7 mmol/L |
| Albumin | 40 g/L |
| Calcium | 2.44 mmol/L |

**Blood results 48 h later:**

| | |
|---|---|
| WCC | $17 \times 10^9$/L |
| Hb | 12.5 g/dL |
| Haematocrit | 0.45 |
| Blood glucose | 9 mmol/L |
| LDH | 445 IU/L |
| AST | 300 IU/L |
| Bilirubin | 67 $\mu$mol/L |
| Creatinine | 130 $\mu$mol/L |
| Urea | 12 mmol/L |
| Albumin | 34 g/dL |
| Calcium | 1.98 mmol/L |

**Arterial blood gas:**

| | |
|---|---|
| pH | 7.30 |
| $PaO_2$ | 8.2 kPa |
| $PaCO_2$ | 4.1 kPa |
| $HCO_3^-$ | 20 mmol/L |
| Base excess | 6 |

**Fluid balance over past 48 h:**

| | |
|---|---|
| Input | 8.3 L |
| Output | 1.7 L |

a. What are the parameters you must use to calculate Ranson's score?
b. Calculate Ranson's score for this patient using the results listed above
c. What is the patient's prognosis?

APACHE, Acute Physiology And Chronic Health Evaluation; AST, aspartate transaminase; CMV, cytomegalovirus; CT, computed tomography; EBV, Epstein–Barr virus; ERCP, endoscopic retrograde cholangiopancreatography; FiO$_2$, fraction of inspired oxygen; Hb, haemoglobin; LDH, lactate dehydrogenase; NSAID, non-steroidal anti-inflammatory drug; PaCO$_2$, partial pressure of arterial carbon dioxide; PaO$_2$, partial pressure of arterial oxygen; SLE, systemic lupus erythematosus; TB, tuberculosis; WCC, white cell count

# EXPLANATION: PANCREATITIS (I)

Acute pancreatitis is defined as an acute inflammatory process of the pancreas with variable involvement of other organ systems. Approximately 20 per cent of patients may develop severe disease, with mortality rates up to 100 per cent. The severity of pancreatitis is often assessed by the following scoring methods (one point for each parameter):

**Ranson's criteria** (usually used for alcohol-induced pancreatitis) **(23a)**:

**On admission:**
- Age >55 years
- WCC >16 × 10⁹/L
- Blood glucose >11 mmol/L
- Blood LDH >400 IU/L
- Blood AST >250 IU/L

**After 48 h of admission:**
- Haematocrit fall >10%
- Blood calcium <2 mmol/L
- Urea rise >10 mmol/L
- $PaO_2$ <8 kPa
- Base deficit >4
- Fluid sequestration >6 L
- Albumin <32 g/L

**Score (23c):**
- 0 to 2 = 2% mortality
- 3 to 4 = 15% mortality
- 5 to 6 = 40% mortality
- 7 to 8 = 100% mortality

**Modified Glasgow criteria**:
$PaO_2$, **A**ge, **N**eutrophil/WCC, **C**alcium, **R**enal function, **E**nzymes: LDH, AST, **S**ugar/glucose.

**APACHE** (Acute Physiology And Chronic Health Evaluation) **II score**: uses age, co-morbidity and 12 physiological parameters to grade the severity of acutely unwell patients. The parameters included are: core temperature, mean arterial pressure, respiratory rate, if $FIO_2$ >50 per cent then record alveolar–arterial gradient, $FIO_2$ <50 per cent then record $PaO_2$, arterial pH, serum [Na⁺], serum [K⁺], serum [creatinine], [haemoglobin], WCC, Glasgow coma score.

A Ranson's or Glasgow score of 3, or APACHE II score of 8, is used as a threshold for diagnosing severe acute pancreatitis and the need for CT assessment and close monitoring for local and systemic complications.

The causes of acute pancreatitis are summarized below:
- Idiopathic (20 per cent of cases)
- Gallstones ⎫
- Ethanol ⎭ 80 per cent of cases
- Trauma
- Steroids
- Mumps and other organisms (EBV, CMV, hepatitis viruses, TB)
- Autoimmune such as SLE
- Scorpion sting/snake bite → *PTH?*
- Hypercalcaemia, hyperlipidaemia, hypotension and hypothermia
- ERCP and post-abdominal surgery
- Drugs: steroids, azathioprine, NSAIDs, furosemide and thiazides
- Other: cystic fibrosis, ischaemia, anatomical variants, e.g. pancreas divisum.

Answers
**21.** F F F T F
**22.** T F T T F
**23.** See explanation for calculating Ranson's score. The score is 8 in this case and is associated with 100 per cent mortality

## 24. Regarding acute pancreatitis

a. It is invariably associated with hyperamylasaemia
b. On examination Grey–Turner's sign (periumbilical ecchymosis) may be present in haemorrhagic pancreatitis
c. Pethidine is not recommended due to spasm of the sphincter of Oddi
d. Surgical management is rarely advisable
e. Measurement of amylase is more sensitive than lipase measurement

## 25. For the following scenarios choose the most appropriate complication. Each option may be used once only

A. Pleural effusions
B. Pancreatic abscess
C. Pancreatic carcinoma
D. Pneumonia
E. Pancreatic necrosis
F. ARDS
G. Renal failure
H. Pancreatic pseudocyst
I. Atelectasis
J. DIC

1. A 45-year-old woman with acute pancreatitis being managed conservatively later develops more severe abdominal pain and a palpable epigastric mass
2. A 50-year-old man admitted with severe epigastric pain radiating to the back develops swinging pyrexia, hypotension, reduced urine output and a tender abdominal mass
3. A 36-year-old patient admitted to ITU with pancreatitis is noted to have petechial skin haemorrhages and bleeding around the venflon site. He has thrombocytopaenia, prolonged prothrombin time and raised fibrin degradation products
4. A patient with pancreatitis develops shortness of breath with increasing oxygen requirements. Chest X-ray shows diffuse alveolar infiltrates

---

ARDS, acute respiratory distress syndrome; CRP, C-reactive protein; CT, computed tomography; DIC, disseminated intravascular coagulation; FBC, full blood count; ITU, intensive therapy unit; IV, intravenous; LDH, lactate dehydrogenase

# EXPLANATION: PANCREATITIS (II)

## ACUTE PANCREATITIS

Patients with acute pancreatitis present with moderate to severe abdominal pain. This is usually diffuse over the **upper abdomen** and may **radiate to the back**. It often persists for hours without relief. The pain may **improve with sitting forwards**. Nausea and vomiting are also common.

On examination, the patient may have epigastric tenderness with or without regional signs of peritonism. **Grey–Turner** (flank ecchymosis) and **Cullen's** (periumbilical ecchymosis) signs may be present in haemorrhagic pancreatitis. These signs are associated with a higher mortality rate.

Investigations should help assess the severity of pancreatitis. These include arterial blood gas analysis (risk of ARDS), blood sampling (FBC, renal profile, liver and bone profile, glucose, amylase, LDH and CRP) and imaging – abdominal ultrasound scan (to exclude gallstones), an erect chest X-ray and abdominal X-ray to exclude other abdominal pathologies such as a perforated peptic ulcer. An abdominal CT scan can help assess severity and complications.

The differential diagnoses of acute pancreatitis include any cause of an acute abdomen such as peptic ulcer disease, acute cholecystitis and intestinal obstruction.

**The majority of cases are managed conservatively** with oxygen therapy, IV fluid resuscitation, analgesia (pethidine is preferred to diamorphine as it is less constipating and causes less sphincter of Oddi spasm) and placement of a nasogastric tube in the presence of an ileus. Antibiotics are reserved for those with confirmed or high suspicion of infection, usually in the setting of severe acute pancreatitis. Surgical management although rarely indicated may be used for certain complications such as pseudocysts, abscesses and infected pancreatic necrosis.

Complications of pancreatitis can be divided into:
- **Local complications**:
  - sterile or infected pancreatic necrosis
  - pancreatic pseudocyst: if asymptomatic, usually treated conservatively, otherwise, radiological, endoscopic or surgical therapy drainage is indicated
  - pancreatic abscess
- **Systemic complications**:
  - respiratory: atelectasis, pleural effusions, ARDS
  - myocardial depression
  - renal failure
  - DIC
  - hyperglycaemia.

Answers
**24.** F F F T F
**25.** 1 – H, 2 – B, 3 – J, 4 – F

## 26. Regarding the features and investigations of chronic pancreatitis

- **a.** The patient may present with diabetes mellitus
- **b.** Constipation is a presenting feature
- **c.** Jaundice can be a presenting complaint
- **d.** Endocrine function tests such as secretin tests may be needed
- **e.** Amylase level is often raised

## 27. Consider management of chronic pancreatitis

- **a.** Pancreatin supplements may cause perianal irritation
- **b.** Antibiotics are indicated
- **c.** In the management of diabetes higher doses of insulin are often required compared with other patients with diabetes
- **d.** Surgery may be indicated
- **e.** Proton pump inhibitors play an important role

CRP, C-reactive protein; CT, computed tomography; ERCP, endoscopic retrograde cholangiopancreatography; FBC, full blood count; MRCP, magnetic resonance cholangiopancreatography; SLE, systemic lupus erythematosus; WHO, World Health Organization

## EXPLANATION: PANCREATITIS (III)

### CHRONIC PANCREATITIS

This is a chronic inflammatory condition characterized by fibrosis, destruction of exocrine and endocrine tissue and chronic pain. Alcohol abuse is the major cause of chronic pancreatitis accounting for 60–70 per cent of cases; 5–15 per cent of cases are idiopathic. Other causes of chronic pancreatitis are cystic fibrosis, obstructive causes such as traumatic strictures and tumours, hereditary pancreatitis, hyperlipidaemia, hyperparathyroidism, SLE, primary biliary cirrhosis and uraemia.

The condition often presents with **chronic upper abdominal pain radiating to the back with associated weight loss**. **Steatorrhoea** (pale bulky oily stool) occurs with <10 per cent lipase secretion. **Diabetes mellitus** occurs with >80–90 per cent gland destruction.

On examination the patient may be cachectic and jaundiced with upper abdominal tenderness ± guarding. Uncommonly, an abdominal mass as a result of a pancreatic pseudocyst may be palpable.

Investigations for chronic pancreatitis include blood tests (FBC, renal profile, liver profile, CRP, amylase and lipase), abdominal X-ray, abdominal ultrasonography, CT scan and if needed MRCP and/or ERCP. Pancreatic function tests for exocrine (faecal elastase-I) and endocrine function (glucose tolerance test) may also be used.

Chronic pancreatitis can be managed as follows:
- **Discontinuation of alcohol**: manage withdrawal with a chlordiazepoxide or diazepam regime
- **Pain management**: use the WHO analgesic ladder and involve the pain team for adequate analgesia. Consider proton pump inhibitors to reduce the risk of peptic ulceration and improve the absorption of pancreatic enzyme supplements. Relieve pancreatic duct obstruction endoscopically with the use of pancreatic stents, pancreatic duct stone removal, or by surgical techniques such as pancreatic resection or the Puestow procedure (longitudinal pancreaticojejunostomy). In refractory cases, consider transcutaneous electrical nerve stimulation and percutaneous or endoscopic ultrasound-guided coeliac plexus block
- **Malabsorption management**: enteric-coated porcine pancreatin supplements. The side-effects of pancreatic enzymes include oral ulceration, perianal irritation, abdominal pain, bowel obstruction, hyperuricaemia and allergic reactions
- **Diabetes management**: note that the diabetes may be brittle if there is insufficient glucagon to counteract hypoglycaemia. Insulin requirements are often lower than in other diabetics.

Pancreatic pseudocyst formation, pancreatic cancer, common bile duct obstruction, duodenal obstruction, peptic ulcer disease and vitamin A, D, E and K deficiency are all potential complications of chronic pancreatitis.

Answers
**26.** T F T F F
**27.** T F F T T

### 28. Risk factors for gallstone disease include

**a.** Total parenteral nutrition
**b.** Older age
**c.** Pregnancy
**d.** Obesity
**e.** Oral contraceptive pill use

### 29. The following patients are at risk of developing gallstones

**a.** A 46-year-old male with a family history of gallstones
**b.** A 33-year-old female with acromegaly, treated with octreotide
**c.** A 35-year-old male who recently lost 12 kg
**d.** A 24-year-old male with beta thalassaemia
**e.** A 57-year-old male who recently had a jejunal resection

### 30. Regarding gallstones

**a.** Diabetes predisposes to gallstone disease by impairing gall bladder emptying
**b.** The majority of gallstones are cholesterol rich
**c.** Haemolytic anaemias predispose to pigment stones
**d.** Pigment stones account for approximately 50 per cent of all gallstones
**e.** 90 per cent are visible on plain abdominal X-ray

### 31. How are gallstones classified? What is the incidence of the different types of gallstones?

## EXPLANATION: GALLSTONES (I)

Gallstones are common and affect more than 20 per cent of patients over the age of 60 years. The risk factors are demonstrated below. The majority of cases are asymptomatic and require no immediate treatment.

**Risk factors for gallstone disease include**:
- Older age
- Female sex
- Family history
- Obesity
- Rapid weight loss
- Pregnancy
- Diabetes mellitus
- Drugs, e.g. oral contraceptives, fibrates, octreotide
- Total parenteral nutrition
- Terminal ileal disease
- Biliary infection.

The pathogenesis of gallstones is attributable in part to **metabolic disturbance of bile**. The Amirand's triangle (see below) demonstrates that changes in bile component increase the risk of lithogenesis.

**Impaired gall bladder emptying** leads to bile stasis as occurs in pregnancy and diabetes. This in turn increases the risk of gallstones. **Bacterial infections** deconjugate bilirubin, which then combines with calcium to form insoluble calcium bilirubinate.

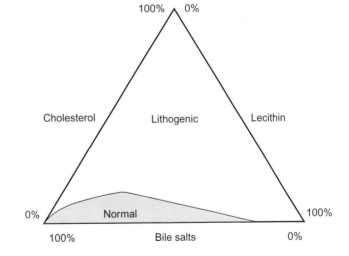

Types of gallstones are **(31)**:
- **Cholesterol-rich stones** (>80 per cent): cholesterol is the major component. They are often multiple and of different sizes. The colour ranges from near white to black
- **Pigment stones** (10 per cent): multiple uniform-sized friable stones, black–brown in colour. They are associated with haemolytic anaemias
- **Mixed stones** (10 per cent ): cholesterol stones accumulate calcium salts including calcium bilirubinate over time. These stones may be visible on plain X-ray.

Answers
**28.** T T T T T
**29.** T T T T T
**30.** T T T F F
**31.** See explanation

**32. A 54-year-old male presents with symptoms of biliary colic. He has no history of gallstone disease**

a. It is the most common presentation of gallstone disease
b. Pain often radiates to the arms in such patients
c. There is a low risk of recurrence
d. Cholecystectomy is contraindicated
e. Ursodeoxycholic acid and a statin should never be co-prescribed

**33. Regarding acute cholecystitis**

a. It may cause local peritonism
b. The presence of fever suggests an alternative diagnosis
c. The patient typically prefers to lie still
d. Boas' sign may be present
e. Antibiotics are of no proven benefit

IV, intravenous; RUQ, right upper quadrant; WCC, white cell count

# EXPLANATION: GALLSTONES (II)

Clinical presentation of gallstone disease depends on the site of gallstone impaction and its complications.

## IN THE GALL BLADDER

- **Biliary colic**:
  - this is the commonest presentation of gallstones. It is caused by the impaction of a stone in Hartmann's pouch or the cystic duct
  - the pain is often localized in the **RUQ or epigastric region**, and may **radiate to the inferior angle of the scapula**. It usually occurs following a fatty meal and may be associated with nausea and vomiting. Acute cholecystitis should be considered if the pain does not settle within 24 h. Differential diagnoses include pancreatitis, oesophagitis and peptic ulcer disease
  - biliary colic is managed conservatively with rehydration, low-fat diet, analgesia and drug dissolution (chenodeoxycholic or ursodeoxycholic acid), with an elective cholecystectomy 6–12 weeks after presentation, as there is a 50 per cent risk of recurrence.
- **Acute cholecystitis**:
  - this is the presence of gall bladder inflammation secondary to chemical irritation, bacterial infection or pancreatic enzyme regurgitation into the biliary system
  - there is a similar presentation as above, but the patient prefers to lie still, and often has signs of inflammation (fever, raised WCC), a positive **Murphy's sign** and possibly **Boas' sign** (hyperaesthesia over right T8 and T9 segments). The patient may be jaundiced if a stone is impacted in the common bile duct
  - treatment includes rehydration, low-fat diet, analgesia, antibiotics and immediate cholecystectomy if the patient does not settle with conservative management. In most cases the cholecystectomy is deferred for 6–12 weeks. It can progress to chronic cholecystitis.
- **Gall bladder mucocele**: a distended gall bladder which is full of clear sterile mucus. This may present with RUQ discomfort or as a RUQ globular mass. It is treated by cholecystectomy.
- **Gall bladder empyema**: this occurs when the cystic duct remains blocked and infection supervenes. The patient presents with symptoms of acute cholecystitis and those of an intra-abdominal abscess such as fever and rigors. Management includes rehydration, analgesia, IV antibiotics, emergency percutaneous cholecystostomy if required, and later cholecystectomy.
- **Gall bladder perforation**: this usually occurs at the fundus (least vascularized area). Patients can present with acute biliary peritonitis or subacutely with a pericholecystitic abscess or cholecystenteric fistula.
- **Gall bladder carcinoma**: a rare, highly malignant neoplasm associated with longstanding gallstone disease, gall bladder polyps and calcified porcelain gall bladders. It is more common in females; 90 per cent are adenocarcinomas. The rich lymphatic and venous drainage of the gall bladder leads to early metastases. Patients with co-existing gallstones are managed with a cholecystectomy. Radiotherapy, chemotherapy and resection with partial hepatectomy are possible management options.
- **Mirizzi's syndrome**: this occurs when a large gallstone in the Hartmann's pouch or cystic duct presses or fistulates into the common bile duct leading to obstructive jaundice. Treatment includes cholecystectomy.

Continued on page 73

Answers
**32.** T F F F F
**33.** T F T T F

**34. For the following scenarios choose the most appropriate complication. Each option may be used once only**

**Options**

A. Obstructive jaundice
B. Biliary colic
C. Gall bladder empyema
D. Acute cholecystitis
E. Gallstone ileus

F. Gall bladder mucocele
G. Acute pancreatitis
H. Gall bladder carcinoma
I. Ascending cholangitis
J. Gall bladder perforation

1. A 49-year-old woman is brought in by ambulance with RUQ and epigastric pain, rigors and a palpable RUQ mass on examination
2. A 42-year-old patient presents with RUQ pain that commenced after a late night meal. On examination the patient had marked tenderness over the RUQ. The patient had a raised CRP and WCC
3. A 50-year-old patient presents with RUQ and shoulder tip pain, jaundice, pruritus and rigors
4. A 56-year-old woman presents with vomiting, generalized abdominal pain and constipation. The abdominal X-ray shows aerobilia
5. A 58-year-old man with known gallstones presents with generalized abdominal pain. On examination he is hypotensive and tachycardic. Abdominal examination reveals a rigid abdomen with no audible bowel sounds

---

CRP, C-reactive protein; ERCP, endoscopic retrograde cholangiopancreatography; IV, intravenous; RUQ, right upper quadrant; WCC, white cell count

## EXPLANATION: GALLSTONES (II) Cont'd from page 71

### IN THE BILIARY TREE

- **Obstructive jaundice**: the patient often presents with a history of biliary-type pain, dark urine, pale stools, pruritus and worsening jaundice.
- **Acute pancreatitis**: stones lying near the ampulla of Vater lead to bile reflux into the main pancreatic duct. Patients present with continuous upper abdominal pain radiating to the back, which may be alleviated by leaning forward.
- **Ascending cholangitis**: bile stasis predisposes to infection, which is characterized by Charcot's triad:
  - rigors
  - obstructive jaundice
  - RUQ pain.
  The infecting organisms include *Escherichia coli*, *Klebsiella*, *Streptococcus* and *Bacteroides* species. Management includes fluid resuscitation, analgesia and IV antibiotics (cefuroxime and metronidazole). If bile duct stones have not passed spontaneously by the time of presentation, ERCP and sphincterotomy or laparoscopic or open stone removal with T-tube drainage are possible options. Elective cholecystectomy is then performed when the acute episode settles.

### OUTSIDE THE BILIARY TREE

- **Gallstone ileus**: this results from a cholecystoduodenal fistula. The gallstone fistulates into the duodenum and enters the gut, resulting in bowel obstruction. Abdominal X-rays classically show aerobilia (air in the bile duct). It is usually managed via an enterotomy. A cholecystectomy with or without biliary reconstruction may be performed.

Answer

**34.** 1 – C, 2 – D, 3 – I, 4 – E, 5 – J

**35. Regarding liver tumours**

    **a.** Hepatic adenomas are the commonest benign hepatic tumours
    **b.** Haemangiomas can be a feature of von Hippel–Lindau disease
    **c.** Use of the oral contraceptive pill is a risk factor for hepatocellular carcinoma (HCC)
    **d.** HCC accounts for 90 per cent of all primary liver tumours
    **e.** HCC is a cause for decompensation in cirrhotic patients

**36. A 63-year-old male with known alcoholic cirrhosis presents with a 6-month history of weight loss, malaise and anorexia. He reports increasing right upper quadrant pain and recent onset of jaundice**

    **a.** What is the prevalence of HCC in the UK? Does the prevalence differ in other parts of the world?
    **b.** List risk factors for HCC
    **c.** What tumour marker could you request in this patient? What is the sensitivity of this investigation?
    **d.** Discuss available management options for patients with HCC

**37. What are hepatic haemangiomas? Which conditions are they associated with?**

AFP, α-fetoprotein; CT, computed tomography; GI, gastrointestinal; HCC, hepatocellular carcinoma; MRI, magnetic resonance imaging

# EXPLANATION: HEPATOBILIARY ONCOLOGY (I)

## BENIGN TUMOURS

Benign tumours are often found incidentally. **Hepatic haemangiomas** are the most common benign hepato-biliary tumours. They are present in 3 per cent of the population. They are masses of blood vessels, which are atypical or irregular in arrangement and size, of unknown aetiology **(37)**. They can occur in Osler–Rendu–Weber syndrome (associated with arterio-venous malformations in the liver, respiratory tract, skin, GI tract and brain), and von Hippel–Lindau disease (autosomal dominant condition associated with renal carcinomas, phaeochromocytoma, retinal and cerebellar haemangioblastomas). This condition is diagnosed with ultrasound and contrast-enhanced CT, where it characteristically has a hypodense centre with ring enhancement of the periphery. Surgical resection is rarely indicated for giant haemangiomas to relieve symptoms or if the diagnosis is in doubt.

**Bile duct adenomas** and **papillomas** are often found incidentally and are small and usually of little clinical importance. **Hepatic adenomas** on the other hand are larger and have the potential to undergo malignant transformation. They are associated with prolonged use of oral contraceptives and pregnancy.

## PRIMARY MALIGNANT TUMOURS

Malignant tumours can be classified as primary or secondary. In the West, the incidence of secondary liver tumours exceeds that of primary tumours; however, in certain regions of the world, for example Southeast Asia, the converse is true.

**Hepatocellular carcinoma (HCC)** is uncommon in the UK, accounting for approximately 2 per cent of all cancers. However, it is the fifth most common cancer in the world **(36a)**. There is a 2–4-fold greater incidence in men. Predisposing factors include hepatitis B and C, cirrhosis secondary to alcohol, and haemochromatosis, aflatoxins and drugs such as anabolic steroids and the oral contraceptive pill **(36b)**.

In patients with cirrhosis, HCC should be suspected during an acute decompensation with, for example, encephalopathy or variceal haemorrhage. HCC is often diagnosed with imaging studies (ultrasound, contrast CT and MRI). Solitary lesions <1 cm in size are difficult to classify. In lesions >2 cm, concomitant finding of two imaging techniques, showing a nodule with arterial hypervascularization, or 1 positive imaging technique and an AFP concentration >400 g/L is highly suggestive of HCC. Note that AFP concentrations are raised in 80 per cent of cases (also raised in testicular or germ cell tumours). Given the sensitivity of AFP measurement for HCC, it is often requested when HCC is suspected **(36c)**.

Management options include **(36d)**:
- **Surgical resection ± liver transplantation**, which is the treatment of choice. This is feasible in <20 per cent of patients
- **Percutaneous methods**, including radiofrequency ablation and ethanol injection
- **Palliative care**, including transarterial embolization and chemoembolization.

Continued on page 77

## Answers

**35.** F T T T T
**36.** See explanation
**37.** See explanation

## 38. Regarding gall bladder cancers

a. They usually present late and hence have a poor prognosis
b. Approximately 5 per cent of cholecystectomy specimens have gall bladder cancer at histology
c. Most are adenocarcinomas and originate in the gall bladder neck
d. They are more common in males
e. Laparoscopic surgical management is a potentially curative option

## 39. Risk factors for gall bladder cancer include

a. A porcelain gall bladder
b. Family history of gall bladder cancer
c. Typhoid carriers
d. A low-fat, high-carbohydrate diet
e. High alcohol consumption

## EXPLANATION: HEPATOBILIARY ONCOLOGY (I)  Cont'd from page 75

**Gall bladder cancer** is the most common biliary tract malignancy. Most gall bladder cancers are found incidentally (1–2 per cent of cholecystectomy cases are found to have cancer at exploration). There is a male:female ratio of approximately 1:4. The peak incidence is between the ages of 70 and 75 years. It is also associated with:

- Gallstone disease
- A porcelain gall bladder
- Gall bladder polyps
- Anomalous pancreaticobiliary duct junction
- Oestrogens
- Cigarette smoking
- High alcohol consumption
- Obesity
- Family history
- Typhoid carriers

Most gall bladder cancers are adenocarcinomas and originate in the gall bladder fundus.

Management options include:

- **Surgery**: a radical cholecystectomy (removal of gall bladder, >2 cm of gall bladder bed and lymph node dissection) ± removal of laparoscopy port sites offers the only curative option. Some centres advocate resection of segments IV and V of the liver
- **Radiotherapy**, which has a place in adjuvant therapy
- **Chemotherapy** using 5-flurouracil and gemcitabine, which has been shown to improve prognosis
- **Palliative care** including:
  - endoscopic or percutaneous transhepatic biliary stenting
  - surgical bypass procedures, e.g. gastrojejunostomy or enteral stenting.

Prognosis is stage dependent with a 40 per cent 5-year survival rate in localized disease and <10 per cent in those with distant disease.

Answers
**38.** T F F F F
**39.** T T T F T

### 40. Regarding cholangiocarcinomas

a. Most are squamous cell carcinomas
b. The majority occur in those aged 40–60 years
c. Ulcerative colitis is a known risk factor
d. Asbestos is a known risk factor
e. The majority arise in the intrahepatic tree

### 41. Regarding pancreatic tumours

a. Diabetes mellitus is a risk factor for pancreatic adenocarcinoma
b. CA 19-9 is a pancreatic tumour marker
c. A Whipple's resection involves resection of the distal stomach, duodenum (D1, D2, D3), common bile duct and pancreas (head, body, tail)
d. Insulinomas are usually metastatic
e. Patients with Zollinger–Ellison syndrome may present with epigastric pain

### 42. Regarding multiple endocrine neoplasia (MEN)

a. It is a group of five syndromes
b. It is inherited in an autosomal dominant pattern
c. Parathyroid tumours are part of MEN I syndrome
d. Phaechromocytoma occur in both MEN IIA and IIB
e. Hyperparathyroidism is the most common initial clinical presentation of MEN I

### 43. A 70-year-old female presents with a 2-month history of dull abdominal pain that radiates to the back. She also reports a 4-month history of diarrhoea, and has dropped a dress size. On examination there is no tenderness on abdominal palpation, and you note a palpable gall bladder

a. What are the common risk factors for this condition?
b. What blood test could you request that would help confirm the diagnosis? What is the sensitivity of this test?
c. Discuss available imaging options to investigate further this patient
d. This patient's condition is not amenable to surgical resection. What management options are available?

### 44. Write short notes on the incidence, classification and management of cholangiocarcinomas

CT, computed tomography; ERCP, endoscopic retrograde cholangiopancreatography; MEN, multiple endocrine neoplasia; MRCP, magnetic resonance cholangiopancreatography; MRI, magnetic resonance imaging

## EXPLANATION: HEPATOBILIARY ONCOLOGY (II)

**Cholangiocarcinoma** is a rare tumour that arises from the epithelium of intrahepatic or extrahepatic bile ducts. More than 90 per cent are adenocarcinomas. Cholangiocarcinoma has an incidence of 1–2 per 100 000 in the UK. Men and women are affected in equal proportions. Two-thirds of all cases occur in populations aged above 65 years **(44)**.

Risk factors for developing cholangiocarcinoma include primary sclerosing cholangitis, ulcerative colitis, congenital biliary cystic disease, biliary parasites and chemicals (asbestos and nitrosamines).

The main aim of curative management is complete tumour resection if possible, and restoration of bile flow. Palliative options include biliary stenting, biliary enteric bypass, photodynamic therapy, chemotherapy and radiotherapy. The median survival in patients receiving only palliative treatment ranges from 2 to 11 months. The median survival for intrahepatic cholangiocarcinoma is 18–30 months, while 5-year survival rates for distal extrahepatic cholangiocarcinoma are 20–30 per cent.

Ninety per cent of **pancreatic cancers** are ductal adenocarcinomas and most cases occur in the head of the pancreas (for endocrine tumours and multiple endocrine neoplasia [MEN] syndromes see summary box on page 80). The male to female ratio is 2:1. The mean age of onset is in the seventh decade. Risk factors for pancreatic cancer are **(43a)**:
- Smoking
- High alcohol consumption
- Diabetes mellitus
- Chronic pancreatitis
- Inherited disorders (MEN, hereditary non-polyposis coli, familial adenomatous polyposis coli, von Hippel–Lindau syndrome).

Patients often present with obstructive jaundice (head of pancreas cancer), pruritus, symptoms of malabsorption, abdominal or back pain and weight loss. They can also present with gastric outlet obstruction (vomiting), venous thrombosis and migratory thrombophlebitis (Trousseau sign). On examination the patient may be cachectic and jaundiced, with a periumbilical mass ± palpable gall bladder. Remember **Courvoisier's law: 'Painless jaundice in the presence of a palpable gall bladder is unlikely to be due to gallstones'**.

Laboratory tests reveal an obstructive jaundice picture in pancreatic head carcinoma. Tumour marker CA 19-9 is raised in approximately 80 per cent of cases **(43b)**, but may also be raised in benign biliary strictures. Imaging studies include ultrasound (percutaneous or endoscopic), CT, MRI/MRCP and ERCP **(43c)**. The latter allows brush cytology, biopsies and palliative stenting.

Continued on page 80

---

Answers
**40.** F F T T F
**41.** T T F F T
**42.** F T T T T
**43.** See explanation
**44.** See explanation

## EXPLANATION: HEPATOBILIARY ONCOLOGY (II)  Cont'd from page 79

Management is as follows:
- **Surgical care**: 20 per cent of patients are amenable to surgical therapy. The major determinant of resectability is the relationship of the tumour to the major vessels (usually the superior mesenteric vein and artery). A Whipple's resection (en bloc removal of distal stomach, duodenum [D1, D2, D3], common bile duct and pancreatic head with gastrobiliary anastomosis) offers a 5-year survival of about 15–20 per cent
- Pancreatic cancer is often resistant to **chemotherapy and radiotherapy**. There is some survival benefit with gemcitabine ± capecitabine **(43d)**
- **Palliative care (43d)**: pain relief (analgesics, TENS, coeliac plexus block and radiotherapy), biliary stenting and enteric bypass procedures such as gastrojejunostomy.

---

**Summary: pancreatic endocrine tumours**
1. Non-functioning tumours
2. Functioning tumours:
   - **insulinoma:** 10 per cent are malignant. Associated with MEN 1. Can present with symptomatic hypoglycaemia secondary to high insulin levels: headache, confusion, motor weakness, ataxia, psychiatric disturbance, convulsions or coma
   - **glucagonoma:** very rare; 80 per cent are malignant. Symptoms similar to diabetes. Often have necrolytic migratory erythema
   - **gastrinoma:** Zollinger–Ellison syndrome is characterized by hypergastrinaemia, and patients with this condition may present with symptoms of peptic ulceration. Fifty per cent are malignant. The tumour can be found in the duodenal wall, pancreas, splenic hilum, mesentery, stomach or ovary
   - **vipoma:** present with profuse watery diarrhoea, dehydration and hypokalaemia
   - **somatostatinoma**
   - **carcinoid tumours.**

---

**Multiple endocrine neoplasia (MEN)** is categorized as shown:
- MEN I: parathyroid adenomas, islet cell tumours, pituitary adenomas
- MEN IIA: medullary thyroid carcinoma, phaeochromocytomas, parathyroid adenomas
- MEN IIB: mucosal neuromas, medullary thyroid carcinoma, phaeochromocytomas.

The liver is the second most common site of **metastatic tumours**. Metastases from the gastrointestinal tract (colorectal, pancreas and gastric), bronchus, breast, ovary and lymphoma are common.

Most tumour deposits are multiple and, with the exception of colorectal metastases, are seldom amenable to resection. However, resection of colorectal liver metastases increases the 5-year survival from 0 per cent to 30 per cent.

---

MEN, multiple endocrine neoplasia; TENS, transcutaneous electrical nerve stimulation

# UPPER GASTROINTESTINAL MEDICINE

# UPPER GASTROINTESTINAL MEDICINE

## 1. Consider dysphagia

a. It is defined as painful swallowing
b. It can occur with pyloric stenosis
c. It can occur with depression
d. Recurrent laryngeal nerve palsy is a known cause
e. It occurs with iron-deficiency anaemia

## 2. Regarding dysphagia

a. A barium meal is the investigation of choice
b. Achalasia is due to the degeneration of the Auerbach's plexus
c. In achalasia, a barium swallow classically reveals a corkscrew appearance
d. Oesophageal dilatation is the first-line treatment for diffuse oesophageal spasm
e. Collagen disorders can present with dysphagia

## 3. A 49-year-old woman presents with shortness of breath and dysphagia. On examination she is pale with no other remarkable findings

a. What other history would you like to elicit?
b. What investigations would you carry out?
c. What are your differential diagnoses?

---

CT, computed tomography; FBC, full blood count; GORD, gastro-oesophageal reflux disease; OGD, oesophago-gastroduodenoscopy

# EXPLANATION: DYSPHAGIA

Dysphagia is defined as **difficulty in swallowing**, while odynophagia is painful swallowing. It is important to distinguish between the two. The aetiology of dysphagia includes **(3c)**:

- **Extraluminal**:
  - retropharyngeal pouch
  - retrosternal thyroid goitre
  - bronchial cancer
  - mediastinal lymphadenopathy
  - paraoesophageal hiatus hernia
  - thoracic aortic aneurysm
  - aberrant subclavian artery (dysphagia lusoria)
- **Intramural**:
  - benign GORD strictures
  - caustic, traumatic and radiotherapy strictures
  - oesophageal cancer
  - achalasia
  - oesophageal web (Plummer–Vinson syndrome) and Schatzki's ring
  - oesophageal diverticula
  - congenital atresia
- **Intraluminal**:
  - foreign body
  - polypoidal tumours
- **Other:** oral (tonsillitis, pharyngitis, epiglottitis, aphthous ulcers), neuromuscular (cerebrovascular accident, motor neuron disease, multiple sclerosis, Parkinson's disease, myasthenia gravis, diabetes, systemic scleroderma) and psychosomatic.

It is important to ascertain the **level of 'sticking'**, the **timing** and the **substrates affected (3a)**. The presence or absence of associated signs and symptoms such as odynophagia, weight loss, dyspeptic symptoms, regurgitation, chronic cough and koilonychia (iron deficiency associated with Plummer–Vinson syndrome) will help reach a diagnosis.

Investigations should include blood analysis (FBC, liver and coagulation profile, renal profile and iron studies), imaging (chest X-ray, barium swallow, CT), endoscopy (OGD) with biopsy, oesophageal manometry and pH studies **(3b)**.

Continued on page 85

Answers

**1.** F F T F T
**2.** F T F F T
**3.** See explanation. c – this patient could coincidentally be anaemic and thus all possible causes of dysphagia should be listed

4. For the following scenarios choose the most appropriate diagnosis. Each option may be
used once only

**Options**

A. Plummer–Vinson syndrome    E. Oesophageal cancer          I. Foreign body
B. Achalasia                  F. Polymyositis               J. Retropharyngeal pouch
C. Thoracic aortic aneurysm   G. Diffuse oesophageal spasm
D. Schatzki ring              H. Systemic sclerosis

1. A 70-year-old man presents with progressive dysphagia, weight loss and voice hoarseness
2. A 26-year-old female presents with intermittent progressive dysphagia and regurgitation of
   fluids. The dysphagia can be overcome by drinking large quantities of water
3. A 75-year-old male presents with a sensation of a lump in the throat, regurgitation of
   food, dysphagia and halitosis
4. A 40-year-old woman complains of dysphagia on swallowing bread and meat. A barium
   swallow reveals barium-coated bread lodged at a narrowing in the lower oesophagus
5. A middle-aged woman presents with dysphagia as well as swollen and stiff fingers. On
   examination she is noted to have calcinosis and telangiectasia

---

OGD, oesophago-gastroduodenoscopy

## EXPLANATION: DYSPHAGIA Cont'd from page 83

### OESOPHAGEAL CONDITIONS

**Achalasia** is a primary peristaltic disorder characterized by failure of relaxation of the lower oesophageal sphincter. It is thought to occur due to the degeneration of Auerbach's plexus. This condition presents between the ages of 20–50 years and affects both sexes equally. Patients present with dysphagia for both solids and liquids (they can present with a worse dysphagia for liquids) and halitosis, as well as sudden cessation of dysphagia when adequate pressure has built up above the obstruction point. Food regurgitation can occur, which may lead to aspiration pneumonia.

A barium swallow shows classical **'bird-beak'** appearance at cardia. There may be no gastric bubble present. An OGD should be performed to exclude malignancy. The cardinal test used to confirm the diagnosis is oesophageal manometry. It reveals failure of lower oesophageal sphincter relaxation and motility.

Management options are:
- **Drug therapy**: nitrates or calcium channel blockers have a direct effect by causing lower oesophageal sphincter relaxation. They may be effective in mild cases
- **Pneumatic balloon dilatation**: there is a 50 per cent success rate, hence it may need to be repeated
- **Endoscopic botulinum toxin injection**
- **Surgical**: Heller's cardiomyotomy involves a longitudinal extramucosal incision.

**Diffuse oesophageal spasm** is characterized by simultaneous contractions of segments of the oesophagus occurring concurrently with normal peristalsis. The patient often presents with retrosternal chest pain (which can mimic cardiac pain) and dysphagia. Barium swallow reveals a characteristic **corkscrew appearance**. Nitrates and calcium channel blockers may provide symptomatic relief. Dilatation or surgical myotomy is indicated in those with severe or persistent symptoms.

**Plummer–Vinson syndrome** often presents in the middle-aged female, with dysphagia and features of chronic iron-deficiency anaemia (shortness of breath, chest pain, koilonychia, angular stomatitis). The dysphagia is a result of a narrowing of the upper oesophagus due to a web projecting from the anterior wall. Endoscopic dilatation is the treatment of choice. Plummer–Vinson syndrome is now seldom seen in clinical practice due to early diagnosis and treatment of iron-deficiency anaemia.

A **Schatzki ring** is a thin mucosal fold found in the lower oesophagus, usually in the presence of a hiatus hernia. The pathogenesis is controversial, both a developmental origin and chronic damage from gastro-oesophageal reflux have been proposed. Asymptomatic Schatzki rings are common, being found in up to 5 per cent of routine barium studies. Patients presenting with symptoms such as food bolus obstruction are treated with endoscopic dilatation.

Answer
**4.** 1 – E, 2 – B, 3 – J, 4 – D, 5 – H

**5. Regarding upper gastrointestinal bleeding**

   **a.** Injection sclerotherapy is the treatment of choice for controlling bleeding gastric fundal varices
   **b.** It can present as unaltered rectal bleeding
   **c.** Mallory–Weiss tears often present with hypovolaemic shock
   **d.** Peptic ulcer disease is the commonest cause
   **e.** Urgent endoscopy is the first line of management as it can be both diagnostic and therapeutic

**6. An 81-year-old woman with a history of recurrent pulmonary emboli and ischaemic heart disease presents with dizziness and shortness of breath over the last 2 days. She has also noticed dark stool. On examination she has a systolic blood pressure of 90 mmHg and heart rate of 72 bpm. She is pale and has cool peripheries. Digital rectal examination reveals melaena**

   **a.** What is your immediate management plan?
   **b.** What in the history may suggest potential high risk of a gastrointestinal bleed?
   **c.** Is she at a high, moderate or low risk of rebleeding?
   **d.** What are the potential causes of melaena?

---

CVP, central venous pressure; ECG, electrocardiogram; FBC, full blood count; GCS, Glasgow coma scale; GI, gastrointestinal; IV, intravenous; NSAID, non-steroidal anti-inflammatory drug; PPI, proton pump inhibitor

## EXPLANATION: GASTROINTESTINAL BLEEDING (I)

This is the most important gastrointestinal emergency, which may present with:
- **Haematemesis**: usually results due to lesions proximal to the ligament of Treitz. It can either be fresh blood or altered 'coffee-ground' blood
- **Melaena**: black tarry offensive stool as a result of bacterial haemoglobin degradation. The bleeding point may be anywhere from the oesophagus to the colon
- **Haematochezia**: fresh per rectal blood. Note that this can also be due to severe upper GI bleeding.

The major causes of **upper GI bleeding** are (6b):
- Peptic ulcer disease
- Gastritis
- Oesophagitis
- Oesophageal and gastric varices
- Oesophageal Mallory–Weiss tear
- Upper gastrointestinal tumours (benign and malignant)
- Drugs: NSAIDs, steroids, aspirin, warfarin
- Aortoduodenal fistula.

Patients with GI bleeding should be assessed with an ABC approach (6a):
- **Protect the airway** if needed and administer high-flow oxygen. Place **large-bore IV cannulae** and draw blood for FBC, renal profile, liver profile, coagulation profile and **cross match for 4–6 units of blood**. Central line access may be required for CVP assessment. Resuscitate with crystalloids initially then colloids as required, and if needed blood. Insert a urinary catheter and monitor urine output. The patient should be kept nil by mouth
- Arrange **urgent endoscopy** in shocked patients or those with known liver disease
- **IV PPI**
- Brief history
- On examination the patient may have signs of hypovolaemic shock (cool and clammy peripherally, tachycardia, hypotension, poor urine output, reduced GCS) and stigmata of chronic liver disease. An abdominal, digital rectal and ECG examination should be performed.

Continued on page 89

Answers
**5.** F T F T F
**6.** a and b – see explanation (page 87), c – Rockall score = 10 and thus high risk of death (page 89), d – see explanation (page 89)

7. Outline the management options for bleeding gastro-oesophageal variceal bleeds

8. Theme – Causes of gastro-oesophageal varices. For the following scenarios choose the most appropriate diagnosis. Each option may be used once only

**Options**

A. Sarcoidosis
B. Right-sided heart failure
C. Hepatitis
D. Budd–Chiari syndrome
E. Portal vein thrombosis

F. Alcoholic cirrhosis
G. Schistosomiasis
H. Tuberculosis
I. Constrictive pericarditis
J. Haemochromatosis

1. A 49-year-old farmer from Egypt presents with ascites and melaena
2. A 34-year-old female smoker, who is on the oral contraceptive pill presents with sudden-onset abdominal pain, nausea, vomiting, tender hepatomegaly and ascites
3. A 46-year-old unemployed, homeless man presents with haematemesis. On examination he is jaundiced with hepatomegaly, splenomegaly and ascites
4. A 16-year-old woman with factor V Leiden deficiency presents with haematemesis. She has a normal liver function tests

GI, gastrointestinal; HR, heart rate; IV, intravenous; sBP, systolic blood pressure

## EXPLANATION: GASTROINTESTINAL BLEEDING (I) Cont'd from page 87

Endoscopy is the investigation of choice in upper GI bleed as it is both diagnostic and therapeutic. It also helps stratify the risk of further bleeding using the **Rockall score**:

|  | Score 0 | Score 1 | Score 2 | Score 3 |
|---|---|---|---|---|
| Age (years) | <60 | 60–79 | ≥80 | – |
| Shock | sBP >100 mmHg<br>HR <100 bpm | sBP >100 mmHg<br>HR >100 bpm | sBP <100 mmHg | – |
| Co-morbidity | None | Cardiac or other major disease | Renal or liver failure | Advanced malignancy |
| Diagnosis | None or Mallory–Weiss tear | All other | Oesophago-gastric malignancy | – |
| Major stigmata of recent bleeding | None or black spots | – | Blood in lumen, clot, non-bleeding visible vessel or spurting bleeding | – |

The Rockall score can also be used to risk stratify patients prior to endoscopy. A total **score of <3 is associated with an excellent prognosis**, while a **score >8 is associated with a high risk of death**.

Common conditions seen in clinical practice include (**6d**):
- **Peptic ulcer**: this often presents with large amounts of coffee-ground vomiting. At endoscopy, possible therapeutic options include injection of adrenaline ± sclerosant into or around the bleeding vessel, laser coagulation and heater probe coagulation
- **Mallory–Weiss tear**: this is a mucosal tear at the gastro-oesophageal junction, which is due to forceful vomiting, retching or coughing. It is often seen after an alcohol binge. The bleeding is usually bright red and self-limiting
- **Gastro-oesophageal varices**: occur as a result of portal hypertension at sites of porto-systemic anastomoses. The causes of gastro-oesophageal varices can be classified as:
  - pre-hepatic: portal vein thrombosis, splenic vein thrombosis
  - hepatic: cirrhosis, hepatitis, granulomatous disease, schistosomiasis
  - post-hepatic: right-sided heart failure, constrictive pericarditis, Budd–Chiari syndrome.

IV telipressin reduces splanchnic blood flow and helps to control bleeding in the acute scenario; IV octreotide is used in some centres. Propranolol is used to lower portal hypertension following stabilization. Endoscopic therapy includes sclerotherapy and variceal banding. Balloon tamponade (Sengstaken tube) can be used as a temporary measure to create haemostasis if bleeding persists (**7**).

Answers

**7.** See explanation
**8.** 1 – G, 2 – D, 3 – F, 4 – E

## 9. Regarding lower gastrointestinal bleeding

a. Patients almost always require surgical management
b. Most patients with Meckel's diverticula present with rectal bleeding
c. Angiodysplasia often presents as painful gastrointestinal bleeding
d. Patients with ischaemic colitis often require bowel resection
e. Labelled red blood cell scan is the investigation of choice for suspected Meckel's diverticulum

## 10. Causes of lower gastrointestinal bleeding include

a. Haemorrhoids
b. Mallory–Weiss tear
c. Diverticular disease

d. Gastric leiomyoma
e. Plummer–Vinson syndrome

## 11. Theme – Gastrointestinal haemorrhage. For the following scenarios choose the most appropriate diagnosis. Each option may be used once only

**Options**

A. Colorectal cancer
B. Mallory–Weiss tear
C. Angiodysplasia
D. Diverticular disease
E. Gastro-oesophageal varices

F. Oesophagitis
G. Ulcerative colitis
H. Haemorrhoids
I. Peptic ulcer disease
J. Ischaemic colitis

1. A 49-year-old man with a high alcohol intake presents with massive haematemesis and signs of shock. On examination he has finger clubbing and gynaecomastia
2. A 55-year-old patient on regular analgesia presents with haematemesis, signs of shock and painless melaena
3. A 69-year-old patient with painless fresh rectal bleeding and no history of weight loss, was noted to have lesions in the ascending colon at colonoscopy which were treated
4. A 36-year-old patient presents with haematemesis after alcohol ingestion and retching
5. A 62-year-old woman presents with fresh rectal bleeding and tenesmus. On defaecation, she passes fresh blood instead of faeces. Furthermore, she has chronic left iliac fossa pain

CT, computed tomography; FBC, full blood count; GI, gastrointestinal; RBC, red blood cell

# EXPLANATION: GASTROINTESTINAL BLEEDING (II)

The major causes of **lower GI bleeding** are:
- Colorectal tumours
- Angiodysplasia
- Inflammatory bowel disease
- Meckel's diverticulum
- Haemorrhoids
- Anal fissures
- Diverticular disease
- Ischaemic colitis.

Resuscitate if necessary as outlined for upper GI bleeding. Massive lower GI bleeding is rare. Investigations should include blood analysis (FBC, renal profile, liver profile, coagulation profile, tumour markers [CEA, CA 19-9]), imaging (abdominal X-ray, barium enema, angiography, 99m-technetium pertechnetate scan if Meckel's diverticulum is suspected, labelled RBC scan for angiodysplasia) and proctoscopy, sigmoidoscopy or colonoscopy ± enteroscopy.

Common causes of lower GI bleed include:
- **Meckel's diverticulum**: this results from an incomplete closure of the ileal end of the vitelline duct. It occurs in 2 per cent of the population, is located 2 feet from the caecum, and is on average 2 inches in length. The condition may present as appendicitis, intussusception or lower GI bleeding due to the presence of gastric mucosa in 40 per cent of cases. Management is by surgical resection
- **Angiodysplasia**: this is a submucosal malformation that usually affects the elderly and is associated with cardiac disease such as aortic stenosis. The commonest site of occurrence is the caecum and ascending colon. It presents with painless fresh rectal bleeding, often in large amounts. It is often managed at colonoscopy with electrocoagulation or by surgical resection
- **Ischaemic colitis**: this condition is more common in elderly patients who have atherosclerotic disease. It is caused by acute or chronic occlusion of the inferior mesenteric artery secondary to atherosclerosis, embolization (from associated atrial fibrillation) or hypovolaemia. Investigations are as above, including an arterial blood gas (may show metabolic acidosis), barium enema (oedema of the mucosa with thumb-printing or stricturing of the colon) and CT scan. Management is usually conservative; bowel resection may be necessary in severe cases.

Answers
**9.** F F F F F
**10.** T F T F F
**11.** 1 – E, 2 – I, 3 – C, 4 – B, 5 – D

## 12. Consider gastro-oesophageal reflux disease

a. It is due to failure of relaxation of the lower oesophageal sphincter
b. Sliding hiatus hernias are more common than the rolling type
c. Sliding hernias have a higher risk of strangulation
d. Ambulatory 24-h pH measurements characteristically show a pH >4 for >40 per cent of the 24-h period
e. Prokinetic agents are contraindicated

GORD, gastro-oesophageal reflux disease; LOS, lower oesophageal sphincter

## EXPLANATION: GASTRO-OESOPHAGEAL REFLUX DISEASE

**Gastro-oesophageal reflux disease (GORD)** is a common condition that affects **more than 30 per cent of the population**. It results from an incompetent lower oesophageal sphincter (LOS). The LOS is a physiological sphincter maintained by the oblique oesophagogastric angle, positive intra-abdominal pressure, diaphragmatic crural sling and mucosal folds at the cardia.

GORD is associated with:
- Smoking
- High alcohol or coffee intake
- Hiatus hernia
- Obesity
- Pregnancy
- Large meals
- Anticholinergics, nitrates and calcium channel blockers
- Post-gastro-oesophageal myotomy.

A hiatus hernia is an abnormal herniation of part of the stomach into the chest cavity. There are two known types:

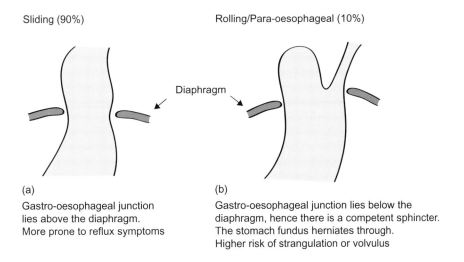

Sliding (90%)

Rolling/Para-oesophageal (10%)

Diaphragm

(a)
Gastro-oesophageal junction lies above the diaphragm. More prone to reflux symptoms

(b)
Gastro-oesophageal junction lies below the diaphragm, hence there is a competent sphincter. The stomach fundus herniates through. Higher risk of strangulation or volvulus

Continued on page 95

Answer
**12.** F T F F F

### 13. Barrett's oesophagus

a. Is the replacement of the normal lower oesophageal columnar epithelium by squamous epithelium

b. Is best diagnosed by a barium swallow

c. Is a pre-malignant condition

d. Is evident in 30 per cent of GORD cases investigated by endoscopy

e. Is best managed by surgery

### 14. What are the pharmacological and non-pharmacological management options for gastro-oesophageal reflux disease?

### 15. The following symptoms in a patient with gastro-oesophageal reflux disease warrant further investigations

a. Weight loss

b. Hoarseness of voice

c. Heart burn

d. Progressive dysphagia

e. Water brash

GORD, gastro-oesophageal reflux disease; OGD, oesophago-gastroduodenoscopy; PPI, proton pump inhibitor

## EXPLANATION: GASTRO-OESOPHAGEAL REFLUX DISEASE  Cont'd from page 93

Clinical features of GORD include:

- Heartburn: described as retrosternal burning pain radiating to the back or epigastric region. The pain is often worse while lying down flat, bending down, straining and after meals. Relief can be obtained with antacids
- Regurgitation of acid: effortless return of gastric contents into the pharynx
- Water brash: acid regurgitation stimulates saliva production
- Dysphagia or odynophagia: possibly due to a stricture
- Atypical symptoms: cough, wheeze and hoarseness following aspiration.

The diagnosis is often clinical. Patients under 40 years are often treated without investigations unless there is associated weight loss, dysphagia, anorexia, haematemesis or melaena, which warrant further investigations. These include OGD and biopsy, barium swallow and biopsy, and ambulatory 24-h pH measures (pH < 4 for more than 40 per cent of a 24-h period).

Management options are **(14)**:

- **Lifestyle modifications** including weight loss, smoking cessation, avoiding precipitants such as alcohol and large meals
- Drug therapy:
  - **antacids** such as magnesium trisilicate (can cause diarrhoea), aluminium hydroxide (can cause constipation) and alginate-containing products (such as gaviscon) can be used after each meal and at bedtime for mild symptoms
  - **H2-receptor antagonists** (such as ranitidine) inhibit acid secretion by acting on parietal cells. They are usually used for mild symptoms
  - **proton pump inhibitors** (such as lansoprazole) inhibit acid secretion by inhibition of the $H^+$–$K^+$/ATPase pump in parietal cells. PPIs are used for refractory cases and severe symptoms
  - **prokinetic agents** (metoclopramide or domperidone) may be used in conjunction with the above therapies
- **Surgical therapy** (open or laparoscopic Nissen fundoplication) may be indicated when medical therapy is symptomatically inadequate; there is a presence of Barrett's oesophagus or atypical symptoms.

Complications of GORD include **oesophagitis** (grade I – erythema, grade II – erosions, grade III – ulcer, grade IV – stricture), **strictures**, **Barrett's oesophagus** (metaplasia of the normal squamous epithelium into columnar epithelium, observed in up to 20 per cent of cases of GORD investigated by endoscopy. Regular surveillance and surgical therapy may be indicated due to the possible progression to malignancy) and **adenocarcinoma**.

---

Answers

**13.** F F T F F
**14.** See explanation
**15.** T T F T F

### 16. Regarding peptic ulcer disease

a. It only occurs in the stomach or duodenum
b. Spicy food may play a role in aetiology
c. It is associated with blood group A
d. Gastric ulcers are more common than duodenal ulcers
e. Herpes simplex infection increases the risk of peptic ulcer disease

### 17. Regarding *Helicobacter pylori* and peptic ulcer disease

a. *H. pylori* is a Gram-negative bacillus
b. *H. pylori* infection should always be eradicated
c. The treatment of *H. pylori* infection involves a triple therapy regime of two anti-acid preparations and an antimicrobial agent
d. Pyloric stenosis may complicate peptic ulcer disease
e. Burns are a risk factor for peptic ulcer disease

### 18. For the following scenarios choose the most likely cause of peptic ulceration. Each option may be used once only

#### Options

A. Alcohol
B. Ibuprofen use
C. Cushing's ulcer
D. Curling's ulcer
E. Zollinger–Ellison syndrome
F. Crohn's disease
G. Hypercalcaemia
H. Chemotherapy
I. Cytomegalovirus
J. Renal failure

1. A 25-year-old rugby player with a recent cruciate ligament tear presents with epigastric pain and haematemesis
2. A 29-year-old woman with a past medical history of resected medullary thyroid cancer is admitted with nausea and severe epigastric pain after meals
3. A 45-year-old patient on the intensive care unit, admitted following major trauma, has a 5 g/dL drop in haemoglobin level and dark stool
4. A 32-year-old man who is non-compliant with highly active antiretroviral therapy presents with abdominal pain and visual disturbance

### 19. What are the surgical management options for peptic ulcer disease? What are the potential complications?

---

CMV, cytomegalovirus; FBC, full blood count; GI, gastrointestinal; NSAID, non-steroidal anti-inflammatory drug; OGD, oesophago-gastroduodenoscopy; PPI, proton pump inhibitor; TB, tuberculosis; VIP, vasoactive intestinal peptide

## EXPLANATION: PEPTIC ULCER DISEASE

Peptic ulcers are defined as breaches of the gastric or duodenal mucosa. Peptic ulceration also occurs in Meckel's diverticulum and around sites of anastomosis such as gastroenterotomies. Duodenal ulcers are more prevalent than gastric ulcers (approximately 4:1 ratio). More than 95 per cent of duodenal ulcers are found on the duodenal cap, while most gastric ulcers are found along the lesser curvature. The aetiological factors include: *Helicobacter pylori* infection (found in 95 per cent of duodenal and 75 per cent of gastric ulcer cases), NSAIDs, smoking, familial, blood group O, renal disease, chemotherapy- or radiotherapy-induced ulcers, Zollinger–Ellison syndrome, hypercalcaemia, granulomatous disease (such as Crohn's disease and sarcoidosis), neoplasia, infections (such as herpes simplex, TB, CMV), severe head injuries (Cushing's ulcer), burns (Curling's ulcer).

Patients can present with **epigastric pain and tenderness**. In duodenal ulcers the pain is worse with fasting and is relieved with food and antacids, while gastric ulcers cause pain that is worse with food and relieved with vomiting. Other forms of presentation include nausea, vomiting, anorexia, weight loss and upper GI bleeding. A succussion splash may be present if there is gastric outlet obstruction.

Investigations should include blood analysis (FBC, renal profile, liver profile and amylase), OGD and antral biopsy for *Helicobacter* status (which also offers therapeutic options). *H. pylori* detection can also be done non-invasively by urease breath test, serology or stool antigen testing.

Management options are:
- **Lifestyle modifications** such as cessation of smoking and NSAIDs
- **Drugs**: simple antacids, $H_2$-receptor antagonists, PPI and *H. pylori* eradication therapy
- **Surgical options (19)**: including selective vagotomy and partial gastrectomy (Bilroth type I or II) are rarely used. A surgical option is indicated when medical therapy recurrently fails, in the presence of complications (such as haemorrhage, perforation or gastric outflow obstruction). Complications of surgery are haemorrhage, reduced gastric emptying, duodenal stump leak, post-vagotomy diarrhoea, early satiety, osteomalacia (vitamin D deficiency), pernicious anaemia and dumping syndrome. Dumping syndrome occurs approximately 30 min after a meal, when the patients experience sweating, palpitations, presyncopal symptoms and abdominal distension. These symptoms occur due to a rapid hyperosmolar load in the jejunum, which results in fluid shift from the vascular compartment, insulin/VIP/neurotensin secretion.

---

*Helicobacter pylori* **infection**

*H. pylori* is a small curved Gram-negative bacillus. More than 70 per cent of infected people are asymptomatic. It is thought to be acquired in early childhood via the faeco-oral or orogastric route. Treatment consists of the use of two antimicrobials in combination with a PPI/bismuth/$H_2$ antagonist, e.g.:
- Lansoprazole, amoxicillin and clarithromycin
- Omeprazole, metronidazole and clarithromycin
- Bismuth-based therapy: which is more effective when co-prescribed with a PPI (quadruple therapy).

---

Answers
**16.** F F F F T
**17.** T F F T T
**18.** 1 – B, 2 – G, 3 – C, 4 – I
**19.** See explanation

## 20. Regarding oesophageal cancers

a. Plummer–Vinson syndrome is a risk factor for adenocarcinoma
b. Achalasia predisposes to squamous cell carcinoma
c. Most squamous cell carcinomas occur in the lower third of the oesophagus
d. Hoarseness of the voice suggests advanced disease
e. Barrett's oesophagus is a risk factor for squamous cell carcinoma

## 21. Consider oesophageal tumours

a. Malignant melanomas can occur in the oesophagus
b. Oesophageal adenocarcinoma predominantly occurs in the lower third of the oesophagus
c. Aspiration pneumonia can be a presenting symptom of oesophageal cancer
d. A clearance margin of 5 cm is the minimum requirement for curative resection of oesophageal cancers
e. Overall 5-year survival of oesophageal cancer is 5 per cent

## 22. Theme – Risk factors for oesophageal tumours. For the following scenarios choose the most appropriate diagnosis. Each option may be used once only

**Options**

A. Darier's disease
B. Coeliac disease
C. Achalasia
D. Malnutrition
E. High nitrosamine intake

F. Tylosis
G. Hiatus hernia
H. Hypothyroidism
I. Plummer–Vinson syndrome
J. Smoking

1. A 65-year-old woman with chronic fatigue, glossitis and koilonychia presents with worsening dysphagia and voice hoarseness
2. A 38-year-old man with a history of yellow hyperkeratosis of his palms and soles was found to have a suspicious oesophageal lesion at routine surveillance endoscopy
3. A 70-year-old man presents to his GP with weight loss and odynophagia. On examination he was thin and unkempt with extensive bruising and corkscrewing of the body hair
4. A 50-year-old patient with a long history of intermittent dysphagia for both solids and liquids presents with anorexia, weight loss and difficulty swallowing saliva

---

CT, computed tomography; FBC, full blood count; GORD, gastro-oesophageal reflux disease; GP, general practitioner

# EXPLANATION: TUMOURS OF THE OESOPHAGUS

Primary tumours of the oesophagus can be divided into benign or malignant. Benign tumours are uncommon and examples include: leiomyomas, lipomas, haemangiomas and squamous papillomas.

Malignant tumours of the oesophagus account for approximately 10 deaths/100 000 population in the UK each year. Oesophageal cancer is more common in men and usually affects individuals over the age of 50 years. The vast majority of malignant tumours are epithelial in origin (squamous cell and adenocarcinoma). However, other uncommon tumours such as carcinoids, malignant melanomas and sarcomas may also occur in the oesophagus.

The incidence of **squamous cell carcinoma** is high in China, Iran and Russia. Risk factors that predispose to squamous call carcinoma include: smoking, alcohol, achalasia, corrosive stricture, high intake of nitrosamines, Plummer–Vinson syndrome, deficiency of vitamins A, C and trace metals, tylosis (a rare autosomal dominant skin condition characterized by hyperkeratosis of the palms and soles).

About 20 per cent of squamous cell carcinomas occur in the upper third of the oesophagus, 50 per cent in the middle and 30 per cent in the lower third. Macroscopically, the tumour may be polypoid, diffusely infiltrative or ulcerated. Microscopically, these tumours are characterized by keratin production and/or prickles.

The incidence of oesophageal **adenocarcinoma** is increasing in the UK, due in part to gastro-oesophageal reflux disease (GORD). Longstanding GORD predisposes to **Barrett's oesophagus**, a condition in which the normal squamous epithelium that lines the distal oesophagus undergoes glandular metaplasia. This may be accompanied by dysplasia which progresses to invasive adenocarcinoma. It is estimated that patients with Barrett's oesophagus are 30–60 times more likely to develop oesophageal adenocarcinoma. Other predisposing factors for this type of tumour include: male gender, obesity and smoking.

Oesophageal cancer may present with progressive dysphagia, weight loss, retrosternal chest pain, a hoarse voice, haematemesis and aspiration pneumonia. These tumours spread by direct extension to local structures (respiratory tree, mediastinum, aorta), through the lymphatic system and via the bloodstream. Patients are investigated by blood analysis (FBC, renal profile, liver and clotting profile), barium swallow, endoscopy and biopsy, endoscopic ultrasound and CT scan. Laparoscopy and thoracoscopy may also be used.

Management options for oesophageal carcinoma are:
- **Curative/surgical**: this is reserved for patients who have disease with no evidence of systemic spread. The main aim of surgery is removal of the oesophagus with at least a 10 cm clearance margin and removal of lymph nodes. An oesophagectomy can be performed by either using a thoracic and abdominal incision (Ivor–Lewis operation) or an abdominal and cervical incision (trans-hiatal operation)
- **Palliative**: There are a number of options which should be tailored to the individual patient and they include stenting, endoscopic dilatation, chemotherapy, radiotherapy, laser therapy, palliative bypass surgery and symptom control.

The overall 5-year survival is about 5 per cent. Survival following surgery is estimated at about 15–20 per cent. Neo-adjuvant radiotherapy and chemotherapy may increase survival rates.

Answers
**20.** F T F T F
**21.** T T T F T
**22.** 1 – I, 2 – F, 3 – D, 4 – C

**23. One of your patients is concerned that he is at high risk of developing gastric cancer. The following are known risk factors**

a. A diet rich in citrus fruit
b. Cigarette smoking
c. Affluence
d. A diet rich in salt
e. A job in the mining industry

**24. Regarding gastric cancer**

a. It is associated with blood type O
b. Pernicious anaemia is a risk factor
c. The overall incidence is increasing worldwide
d. It is twice as common in males as in females
e. Most lesions occur in the gastric cardia

**25. Consider gastric tumours**

a. Leiomyomas have a classical volcano-like appearance at endoscopy
b. Malignant tumours are usually cured by partial gastrectomy
c. Trousseau's sign is the presence of a prominent left supraclavicular lymph node associated with gastric cancers
d. They can metastasize to the ovaries
e. The superficial spreading variant is associated with a better prognosis

**26. A 65-year-old woman presents with symptoms suggestive of gastric carcinoma**

a. How does gastric cancer typically present? Is it generally diagnosed early or late in the course of the disease?
b. How would you further investigate this patient?

The results of your investigations confirm that your patient has a small tumour confined to the fundus

c. How would you manage this patient?
d. The patient and her family are keen to discuss prognosis. How would you counsel this patient?

## EXPLANATION: TUMOURS OF THE STOMACH

Benign gastric tumours are detected in about 1–2 per cent of patients undergoing endoscopy. They include hyperplastic polyps, adenomas and leiomyomas.

The majority (>90 per cent) of malignant gastric tumours are **adenocarcinomas**. A small proportion of malignant tumours are lymphomas, carcinoids and stromal cell tumours. Gastric carcinoma affects about 15/100 000 people in the UK. Higher incidence rates are found in countries such as Japan, Chile and Scandinavia. However, the overall incidence in the Western world has decreased over the last 50 years, possibly as a result of a decline in the prevalence of *Helicobacter pylori* infection rates and improved methods of food preservation. Gastric carcinoma is **twice as common in men as in women** and has a peak incidence in the fifth decade. Several environmental and genetic factors have been implicated in the aetiology of gastric carcinoma.

Risk factors for gastric carcinoma include:
- **Dietary and environmental factors**: high-nitrite diet, smoked/salted foods, cigarette smoking, lack of fresh fruit and vegetables, workers in mining and rubber industries, low social class
- **Gastric pathology**: gastric adenomas, pernicious anaemia, chronic atrophic gastritis, intestinal metaplasia, previous gastric surgery, *Helicobacter pylori* infection
- **Genetic**: blood group A, positive family history.

Approximately **50 per cent of gastric carcinomas occur in the gastric antrum**, 25 per cent in the cardia, and the remainder in the body. They can be classified as early or advanced. Early gastric carcinoma is defined as tumours restricted to the submucosal layer, whilst advanced carcinoma refers to tumours that have penetrated the muscular layer. Macroscopically, four pathological types are recognized: ulcerative, polypoid, linitis plastica (a diffusely infiltrative tumour type which may produce a 'leather-bottle' appearance), superficial spreading.

Early gastric carcinoma is often asymptomatic. As a result, the disease often presents late with dyspepsia, dysphagia, anorexia, vomiting, weight loss and haemorrhage **(26a)**. On examination patients may have cachexia, an epigastric mass, hepatomegaly, jaundice, ascites, Troiser's sign (enlarged left supraclavicular lymph node – Virchow's node) and paraneoplastic manifestations such as acanthosis nigricans.

Gastric cancer can spread by direct invasion into local structures, via the lymphatics, haematogeneously and by transcoelomic spread. Investigations are similar to those for oesophageal cancer **(26b)**.

Management options **(26c)** are:
- **Curative/surgical**: surgical resection is the only potentially curative therapy. A total gastrectomy is usually the procedure of choice. Partial gastrectomies may be adequate for tumours in the distal two-thirds of the stomach. Oesophagogastrectomy is reserved for gastro-oesophageal junctional and cardia tumours. A 5 cm clearance margin is required. Following surgery, the 5-year survival rate for tumours confined to the stomach with no nodal spread is 30–50 per cent. The 5-year survival rate drops to 10 per cent in more advanced disease **(26d)**.
- **Palliative**: the options include palliative resection or bypass, chemotherapy and symptom control.

Answers
**23.** F T F T T
**24.** F T F T F
**25.** T F F T T
**26.** See explanation

### 27. The following are causes of malabsorption

a. Chronic pancreatitis
b. Neomycin therapy
c. Post-Whipple's procedure
d. Whipple's disease
e. Left hemicolectomy

### 28. Match the following patients with the vitamin deficiencies listed below. Each option may only be used once

**Options**

A. Vitamin A deficiency
B. Vitamin $B_{12}$ deficiency
C. Vitamin C deficiency
D. Iron deficiency
E. Vitamin D deficiency
F Vitamin K deficiency
G. Protein deficiency

1. A young child who has become increasingly weak, and has generalized oedema
2. A middle-aged woman who complains of night blindness and dry eyes
3. A young woman with spoon-shaped nails and a smooth red tongue
4. A young vegan who presents with numbness of the feet and hands
5. A teenager with gingivitis and an acutely painful, swollen knee

CRP, C-reactive protein; ESR, erythrocyte sedimentation rate; FBC, full blood count; GI, gastrointestinal

## EXPLANATION: SMALL-BOWEL DISORDERS (I)

**Malabsorption** is defined as a failure of absorption of nutrients from the GI tract. It can be classified either as specific malabsorption (the malabsorption of a specific nutrient such as vitamin $B_{12}$ in pernicious anaemia) or generalized malabsorption.

There are two main sites of nutrient absorption in the small intestine. The **duodenum and jejunum** are responsible for the absorption of glucose, folic acid, iron, ascorbic acid, protein and fat, including fat-soluble vitamins (vitamin A, D, E and K), pyridoxine and riboflavin. The **terminal ileum** is the site of absorption of bile salts and vitamin $B_{12}$.

Causes of malabsorption include:
- **Small intestinal pathology**: coeliac disease, Crohn's disease, giardiasis, tropical sprue, Whipple's disease, small-bowel resection, mesenteric ischaemia, bacterial overgrowth
- **Biliary pathology**: obstructive jaundice, drugs such as cholestyramine
- **Pancreatic pathology**: chronic pancreatitis, cystic fibrosis, pancreatic cancer
- **Other**: thyrotoxicosis, drugs such as neomycin.

Clinical features may include:
- **General**: weight loss, malaise, growth retardation in children, diarrhoea, abdominal distension
- **Protein deficiency**: muscle weakness, subcutaneous fat loss, oedema
- **Fat malabsorption**: dry eyes and night blindness (vitamin A), bone pain, proximal myopathy and osteomalacia (vitamin D), coagulopathy (vitamin K)
- **Iron and folate deficiency**: pallor, koilonychia, angular stomatitis, atrophic glossitis
- **Vitamin B deficiency**: diarrhoea, dermatitis, peripheral neuropathy and dementia
- **Vitamin C deficiency**: gingivitis, loose teeth, halitosis, corkscrew hair, bleeding into the gums or joints.

Investigations often used are blood analysis (FBC, renal profile, bone profile, liver profile, clotting profile, CRP, ESR, vitamin $B_{12}$, folate, ferritin levels, trace elements, anti-gliadin and anti-endomyseal antibodies), gastroscopy and duodenal biopsy, hydrogen breath tests, small-bowel follow-through or CT enteroclysis and faecal elastase-1 (a test for exocrine pancreatic insufficiency).

Continued on page 105

Answers
**27.** T T T T F
**28.** 1 – G, 2 – A, 3 – D, 4 – B, 5 – C

## 29. Coeliac disease

a. Is invariably diagnosed in infancy
b. Is the commonest cause of malabsorption worldwide
c. Is associated with HLA DQ2
d. Affects the whole of the small intestine
e. The gold-standard investigation is detection of anti-endomyseal antibodies

30. You are the new F1 doctor on an upper GI firm. Your consultant asks you to attend his outpatients' clinic, where you are assigned several patients to see. The first patient is a 33-year-old woman from Dublin, who complains of longstanding diarrhoea, malaise and an itchy rash on her elbows and knees

a. What condition do you suspect this patient may have? What patient characteristics would fit with your diagnosis?
b. What simple investigations would lend weight to your presumptive diagnosis? How do you make a definitive diagnosis?
c. How would you initially manage this patient's GI and dermatological symptoms? If the patient fails to respond, what further treatment is indicated?

GI, gastrointestinal; HLA, human leucocyte antigen; Ig, immunoglobulin

## EXPLANATION: SMALL-BOWEL DISORDERS (I)  Cont'd from page 103

### COELIAC DISEASE

Coeliac disease is an autoimmune condition in which exposure to **α-gliadin** (gluten component) causes villous atrophy and subsequently malabsorption. It is the most common cause of malabsorption in the Western world and has a high prevalence in Ireland (1 in 150). There is a slightly higher preponderance in females. There are strong HLA associations, especially with **HLA DQ2**. There are two peaks in incidence; infancy and between the ages of 30 and 40 years.

The disease mainly affects the proximal small bowel and is characterized by partial or complete villous atrophy, damage to the epithelial cells and brush border. There is also mucosal thickening as a result of chronic inflammation.

Patients are often asymptomatic, but can present with features of malabsorption and dermatitis herpetiformis, which is an uncommon pruritic vesicular rash usually found on the elbows, knees and buttocks associated with coeliac disease **(30a)**.

Investigations often show micro or macrocytic anaemia. **Anti-endomyseal/anti-gliadin/anti-reticulin/anti-transglutaminase antibodies** are raised unless the patient has selective IgA deficiency (present in 2.5 per cent of coeliac disease patients). Diagnostic tests include endoscopic jejunal biopsy and test response to a gluten-free diet **(30b)**.

Management includes implementing a gluten-free diet (avoid wheat and barley, however, gluten in rice, maize and soya can be eaten) with iron and folate supplements. Corticosteroids can be used for severe cases. Dapsone may be beneficial for dermatitis herpetiformis **(30c)**.

Coeliac disease may be complicated by osteoporosis, ulcerative jejunitis, small-bowel strictures, lymphoma and oesophageal carcinoma.

Answers

**29.** F F T F F
**30.** See explanation

### 31. Regarding bacterial overgrowth

a. Achlorhydria is a risk factor
b. Systemic sclerosis is a risk factor due to increased intestinal motility
c. It may present with symptoms of vitamin $B_{12}$ deficiency
d. The Schilling test may be useful in diagnosis
e. Antibiotics should not be prescribed as they may worsen the condition

### 32. Theme – Causes of malabsorption. For the following scenarios choose the most appropriate diagnosis. Each option may be used once only

**Options**

A. Giardiasis
B. Cystic fibrosis
C. Chronic pancreatitis
D. Crohn's disease
E. Ulcerative colitis

F. Whipple's disease
G. Coeliac disease
H. Blind loop syndrome
I. Gastroparesis
J. Tropical sprue

1. A 35-year-old man presents with steatorrhoea, abdominal pain, fever and weight loss. Small-intestinal biopsy reveals stunted villi with PAS-positive macrophages
2. A 24-year-old patient presents with intermittent diarrhoea, right iliac fossa pain, weight loss and a macrocytic anaemia
3. A 60-year-old man with a history of epigastric pain radiating to the back, and oily bulky offensive stool that is difficult to flush away
4. A 33-year-old Irish female with diarrhoea, weight loss and angular stomatitis who has noted that her symptoms improve with omission of bread from her diet
5. A 58-year-old man with known diabetic neuropathy presents with increasing weight loss and diarrhoea. He was noted on routine blood analysis to have a macrocytic anaemia

---

PAS, periodic acid–Schiff

# EXPLANATION: SMALL-BOWEL DISORDERS (II)

## BACTERIAL OVERGROWTH/BLIND LOOP SYNDROME

The proximal small intestine normally contains $<10^4$ colony-forming units per mL of aspirate, due in part to the effects of gastric acid, peristalsis and local immune defence mechanisms. The terminal ileum contains $10^5$ to $10^9$ faecal-type organisms, which are beneficial in the synthesis of folate and vitamin K. However, in excess these organisms are detrimental as they deconjugate bile salts and metabolize vitamin $B_{12}$.

Any situation in which gastric acid secretion is reduced (achlorhydria), or intestinal motility is impaired (e.g. systemic sclerosis), may lead to bacterial overgrowth. Anatomical disorders that result in stagnation of intestinal contents (such as jejunal diverticulosis), or seeding of the proximal small intestine with colonic-type bacteria (fistulating Crohn's disease) also predispose to abnormal bacterial proliferation.

The condition presents with **diarrhoea, steatorrhoea and vitamin $B_{12}$ deficiency**. The diagnosis can be supported using breath tests (hydrogen breath test and $^{14}$C-glycocholate breath test), analysis of small-intestinal aspirate and the Schilling test.

Treatment should be aimed at correcting the underlying cause if possible. Rotating courses of antibiotics such as metronidazole or tetracycline may be beneficial.

## TROPICAL SPRUE

Tropical sprue is a chronic diarrhoeal disease of likely infectious origin that involves the small intestine and is characterized by malabsorption of nutrients, especially folic acid and vitamin $B_{12}$. The aetiology of this condition is unclear, but it occurs in residents or visitors to certain countries in the tropics. Duodenal biopsies show similar features to untreated coeliac disease. Treatment is with broad-spectrum antibiotics such as tetracycline, together with folic acid for 3–6 months.

## WHIPPLE'S DISEASE

This is a rare disease that has a male predominance, caused by infection with *Tropheryma whipplei*. It presents with arthralgia, steatorrhoea, fever, lymphadenopathy and sometimes there may be heart, lung or brain involvement. The villi are stunted and contain PAS-positive macrophages on histology. It responds to a prolonged course of treatment with antibiotics such as cotrimoxazole.

Continued on page 109

Answers
**31.** T F T T F
**32.** 1 – F, 2 – D, 3 – C, 4 – G, 5 – H

## 33. Regarding carcinoid

a. Patients can present with Cushing's syndrome
b. Carcinoid tumours are always malignant
c. 24-h urine collection for 5-HIAA may be useful in diagnosis
d. Octreotide is a possible treatment option
e. It may occur in the ovary or testis

## 34. Regarding lymphoma

a. The large bowel is the most common site of extra-nodal disease
b. MALT (mucosa-associated lymphoid tissue) lymphoma is associated with *Helicobacter pylori* infection
c. Patients often present non-specifically
d. Mediterranean lymphoma has an excellent prognosis
e. Radiotherapy is contraindicated

---

ACTH, adrenocorticotrophic hormone; CT, computed tomography; GI, gastrointestinal; 5-HIAA, 5-hydroxy indole-acetic acid; 5-HT, 5-hydroxytryptamine; MALT, mucosa-associated lymphoid tissue; MIBG, [131]iodine-meta-iodobenzylguanidine

## EXPLANATION: SMALL-BOWEL DISORDERS (II) Cont'd from page 107

### SMALL-BOWEL TUMOURS

Small-bowel tumours are rare. Benign tumours include small stromal tumours and adenomas. Malignant tumours include carcinoid, lymphoma, adenocarcinoma and leiomyosarcoma.

**Carcinoid** is a neoplasm of the gastrointestinal neuroendocrine cells capable of producing 5-HT. It is more common in the appendix and terminal ileum; however, it may occur anywhere in the GI tract as well as in the bronchi, ovary or testis. Carcinoid tumours may be benign and the malignant potential depends on:
- **Size**: there is a 70 per cent chance of metastases if the tumour is >2 cm in diameter
- **Site**: carcinoid tumours originating in the ileum, stomach and colon have a higher potential of malignancy compared to those in the appendix and rectum
- **Depth of invasion**: there is a 90 per cent incidence of metastases if there is >50 per cent invasion through the wall.

Patients can present with abdominal pain, GI obstruction or intussusception, GI bleeding, appendicitis, Cushing's syndrome due to ectopic ACTH secretion, carcinoid syndrome or carcinoid crisis. Carcinoid syndrome occurs in 5–10 per cent of patients, who have hepatic metastases. The patients present with facial and neck flushing, profuse colicky diarrhoea, weight loss, wheeze and right-sided heart failure due to fibrosis of pulmonary or tricuspid valves.

Patients can be investigated with 24-h urine collection for 5-HIAA (metabolite), chest X-ray, liver ultrasound scan, chest/abdomen/pelvis CT scans, somatostatin receptor scintigraphy (octreoscan) and MIBG nuclear medicine scans.

Patients can be treated medically with octreotide (somatostatin analogue) or interferon-α. Surgical resection of tumours and embolization of hepatic metastases are an option. The median survival is 5–10 years.

In **lymphoma** the small bowel is the commonest site of extra-nodal disease. Lymphomas are most commonly found in the ileum. There are three main types:
- MALT (mucosa-associated lymphoid tissue) lymphoma: B-cell lymphoma. Associated with *Helicobacter pylori* infection
- Sprue-associated lymphoma: T-cell lymphoma associated with coeliac disease
- Mediterranean lymphoma: B-cell lymphoma with poor prognosis.

Patients present with non-specific symptoms such as abdominal pain, diarrhoea, weight loss, abdominal masses and lymphadenopathy. Most patients are managed with surgery and radiotherapy. Extensive tumours may require additional chemotherapy.

Answers
**33.** T F T T T
**34.** F T T F F

## 35. Regarding Crohn's disease

**a.** Bloody diarrhoea is a common presentation
**b.** It usually involves both small and large bowel
**c.** Smoking is protective
**d.** There is a higher risk of anorectal complications than ulcerative colitis
**e.** Corticosteroids are preferable to sulfasalazine for remission maintenance

## 36. The following features are more consistent with Crohn's disease than ulcerative colitis

**a.** Crypt abscesses at histology
**b.** Cobblestone appearance at colonoscopy
**c.** Depletion of goblet cells at histology
**d.** Granulomata at histology
**e.** Rose thorn appearance at radiology

## EXPLANATION: INFLAMMATORY BOWEL DISEASE (I) – CROHN'S DISEASE

Crohn's disease is a chronic inflammatory disease of the gastrointestinal tract affecting any part of the tract from the mouth to the anus, as well as having extra-intestinal features. Most cases affect the small and large bowel, especially **the ileocaecal region**. In about 45 per cent of cases there is small and large bowel involvement. The disease is limited exclusively to the small bowel or large bowel in 30 per cent and 20 per cent of cases, respectively. The aetiology remains unknown, but many factors have been considered including infectious agents such as mycobacteria and measles, diet, smoking, cytokine-mediated damage and genetics (mutation in the *CARD15* gene).

### PATHOLOGICAL FEATURES

**Macroscopic appearances**:
- the bowel has a hyperaemic appearance
- thick fibrotic bowel wall (lead-pipe appearance)
- skip lesions
- presence of adhesions
- thick and corrugated mesentery
- presence of fistulae
- mucous membrane is red, aphthous ulcerations present with cobblestone appearance
- the rectum is normal in 50 per cent of cases

**Microscopic findings**:
- transmural inflammation
- cryptitis ± crypt abscesses with polymorphs
- granulomas.

One-third of patients present before the age of 20 years. It is more common in northern European and Jewish populations. Common presentations include **(38a)**:
- Recurrent right lower quadrant pain
- Diarrhoea. Distal colitis would lead to mucus and pus defaecation. The patient may have steatorrhoea due to reduced bile salt absorption
- Fever
- Weight loss
- Gross per rectal bleeding is not as common as in ulcerative colitis
- Perianal fissures, fistulas and abscesses
- Pneumaturia
- Extra-intestinal manifestations such as vitamin $B_{12}$ deficiency, osteomalacia, finger clubbing, erythema nodosum, pyoderma gangreonosum, aphthous stomatitis, arthropathy, anterior uveitis, primary sclerosing cholangitis and amyloidosis **(38b)**.

Examination may be unremarkable. The extra-intestinal manifestations listed above may be evident. On abdominal examination, the patient may have a tender right iliac fossa or a mass palpable. Digital rectal examination may reveal fissures, fistulas and perianal abscesses.

Continued on page 113

Answers
**35.** F T F T F
**36.** F T F T T

**37. Regarding the management of Crohn's disease**

a. In young patients, nutritional therapy alone may achieve remission in up to 80 per cent of cases
b. Antibiotics such as metronidazole are of little benefit, except in the presence of suppurative complications
c. Less than a quarter of patients require some form of surgical intervention
d. Antimotility drugs are useful in the control of diarrhoea
e. Infliximab may worsen severe disease

**38. A 23-year-old male presents with a possible diagnosis of Crohn's disease. You are the admitting junior doctor in the emergency department and are asked to clerk this patient**

a. How does Crohn's disease typically present? Is per rectal bleeding common?
b. On examination you note finger clubbing. What other examination findings are you likely to find?
c. Although you strongly suspect Crohn's disease, what other conditions can present in a similar manner?
d. How would you investigate this patient?

Armed with the results of your investigations, you confidently diagnose Crohn's disease

e. Discuss the available management options for this patient

CRP, C-reactive protein; CT, computed tomography; ESR, erythrocyte sedimentation rate; FBC, full blood count; Ig, immunoglobulin; MRI, magnetic resonance imaging

## EXPLANATION: INFLAMMATORY BOWEL DISEASE (I) – CROHN'S DISEASE Cont'd from page 111

Investigations should include blood analysis (FBC, CRP, ESR, renal profile, liver profile, blood cultures, iron studies, folate level and vitamin $B_{12}$ level), stool microscopy and culture, abdominal X-ray, small-bowel enema (may reveal fistulae, strictures, string sign of Kantor – string of sausages appearance, rose-thorn mucosal appearance), endoscopy and biopsy as well as CT scan (MRI scan for pelvic lesions) **(38d)**.

Differential diagnoses include ulcerative colitis, diverticular disease, tuberculosis, *Yersinia* ileitis, intestinal lymphoma, carcinoma, carcinoid and actinomycosis **(38c)**.

**Management** options include the following **(38e)**:
- In young patients with active Crohn's disease, **primary nutritional therapy** with elemental and/or poly-meric formula taken by mouth or nasogastric tube for 4–6 weeks achieves remission in 50–80 per cent of patients. An alternative for steroid-resistant or steroid-refractory disease is total parenteral nutrition. Avoid antimotility drugs such as codeine and loperamide as they can precipitate paralytic ileus and megacolon
- **Aminosalicylates**: mesalazine (Asacol, Pentasa) has a role both in active disease and in maintenance of remission. They are first-line therapy in mildly active disease
- Antibiotics such as **metronidazole** have a modest benefit in Crohn's colitis and fistulating disease even in the absence of suppurative complications
- **Prednisolone** is beneficial in active disease
- **Immunosuppressive agents** (azathioprine, 6-mercaptopurine, methotrexate, ciclosporin) are used in cases where remission is difficult to achieve
- **Infliximab** (IgG antibody to tumour necrosis factor) is used for patients who are refractory to other treatments
- **Surgical management**: as many as one-half of patients with Crohn's disease will need some form of surgical intervention. The indications are cases refractory to medical treatment, the presence of fistulae, perianal disease and strictures causing mechanical bowel obstruction.

The mortality associated with Crohn's disease is twice that of age-matched controls. There is 100-fold greater risk of small- or large-intestinal adenocarcinoma.

Answers

**37.** T F F F F
**38.** See explanation (pages 111 and 113)

**39. Regarding ulcerative colitis**

    **a.** It usually does not affect the small bowel
    **b.** It has a higher risk of colorectal cancer than Crohn's disease
    **c.** CRP is a marker used in the assessment of severity
    **d.** Toxic dilatation (defined as colonic diameter $>10$ cm) is a known complication
    **e.** Barium enema is an important investigation during an acute severe attack

**40. Ulcerative colitis is associated with the following extra-intestinal manifestations**

    **a.** Primary sclerosing cholangitis
    **b.** Dermatitis herpetiformis
    **c.** Erythema nodosum
    **d.** Splinter haemorrhages
    **e.** Episcleritis

**41. When grading the severity of ulcerative colitis**

    **a.** Fewer than four episodes of diarrhoea per day suggests mild disease
    **b.** A haemoglobin level of less than 10.6 g/dL indicates moderate disease
    **c.** The presence of any rectal bleeding suggests moderate or severe disease
    **d.** Low-grade pyrexia may be present in mild disease
    **e.** Tachycardia indicates severe disease

**42. Construct a table listing the key clinical, radiological and histological differences between Crohn's disease and ulcerative colitis**

---

CRP, C-reactive protein; ESR, erythrocyte sedimentation rate

## EXPLANATION: INFLAMMATORY BOWEL DISEASE (II) – ULCERATIVE COLITIS

Ulcerative colitis is a **chronic inflammatory disease of the colonic mucosa**. In 50 per cent of cases it is limited to the rectum and rectosigmoid region. About 20 per cent have a total colitis. Ulcerative colitis primarily affects those between the age of 20 and 40 years; 10–20 per cent of patients have a positive family history. Like Crohn's disease, the aetiology remains unknown.

### PATHOLOGICAL FEATURES

**Macroscopic appearances**
- hyperaemic and oedematous mucosa
- inflammatory pseudopolyps may be present
- continuous distribution
- deep punctuate ulcerations
- strictures and fistulae are rare

**Microscopic appearances**
- limited to mucosa
- no granulomata
- gland destruction
- crypt abscesses.

### CLINICAL FEATURES

- Rectal bleeding is a hallmark of ulcerative colitis
- Diarrhoea is not always present; it may be mixed with blood, mucus or pus
- Abdominal pain is not usually a prominent feature. When present it is usually lower abdominal or left iliac fossa pain
- Urgency and abdominal cramps prior to defaecation
- Anorexia
- Weight loss
- Fever
- Extraintestinal features are similar to those in Crohn's disease with an additional association with ankylosing spondylitis.

Investigations are similar to those for Crohn's disease. Barium studies reveal a loss of haustral patterns, lead-pipe colon and a collar-stud appearance due to the punctate ulcers.

The table below summarizes the **grading of ulcerative colitis**:

|  | Mild cases | Moderate cases | Severe cases |
|---|---|---|---|
| Episodes of diarrhoea | ≤3/day | 4–6/day | ≥7/day |
| Rectal bleeding | Small amounts | Moderate | Profuse |
| Temperature | Normal | 37.1–37.8 °C | >37.8 °C |
| Heart rate | <70 bpm | 70–90 bpm | >90 bpm |
| Haemoglobin level | >11 g/dL | 10.5–11 g/dL | <10.5 g/dL |
| ESR | <30 mm/h | <30 mm/h | >30 mm/h |

Continued on page 116

Answers
**39.** T T F F F
**40.** T F T F T
**41.** T T F F T
**42.** See explanation (page 116)

## EXPLANATION: INFLAMMATORY BOWEL DISEASE (II) – ULCERATIVE COLITIS
### Cont'd from page 115

Differential diagnoses include infection such as *Clostridium difficile* diarrhoea, Crohn's disease, ischaemic or radiation colitis.

### MANAGEMENT

- **Dietary management** as for Crohn's disease.
- For mild and moderate attacks the patient should be **nil by mouth** and receive IV rehydration. In proctitis it is reasonable to use topical mesalazine (suppository or foam enema). Otherwise high-dose **mesalazine or prednisolone** is commenced. Aminosalicylates are used to maintain remission.
- For severe attacks the patient should also be nil by mouth and receive IV fluids. **Thromboprophylaxis** should be given. IV steroids (hydrocortisone) are instituted. Consider **ciclosporin or azathioprine** for refractory disease.
- Indications for **surgery** (colectomy with temporary ileostomy and ileoanal pouch construction) are severe attacks unresponsive to medical therapy, the presence of complications such as perforation, haemorrhage, toxic megacolon (colonic diameter >6 cm), high-grade dysplasia and colonic cancer. Chronically active disease adversely affecting quality of life may also be managed surgically.

Eighty per cent have relapse-remitting disease, while 10 per cent have a chronic continuous course. There is a higher incidence of malignancy than in Crohn's disease.

The key differences between Crohn's disease and ulcerative colitis are shown below (42):

| | Crohn's disease | Ulcerative colitis |
|---|---|---|
| Clinical features | Mouth to anus | Large bowel affected |
| | Bloody diarrhoea uncommon | Bloody diarrhoea common |
| | Abdominal mass common | Abdominal mass uncommon |
| | Perianal disease common | Perianal disease uncommon |
| | Rectal involvement uncommon | Rectal involvement usual |
| Radiological features | Segmental regions affected | Continuous distribution |
| | Rose-thorn appearance | Collar-stud appearance |
| | Strictures common | Strictures uncommon |
| | Fistulae common | Fistulae uncommon |
| Histological features | Transmural involvement | Mucosal involvement |
| | Skip lesions | Continuous areas affected |
| | Glands preserved | Glands destroyed |
| | No polyps | Pseudopolyps |
| | Thickened bowel wall | No thickening of bowel wall |
| | Granulomata | No granulomata |
| | | Crypt abscesses more common |
| | | Depleted goblet cells |
| | | Malignancy more common |

IV, intravenous

# LOWER GASTROINTESTINAL MEDICINE

### 1. Regarding diverticular disease

a. It most commonly affects the rectum
b. Diverticula can be discovered incidentally in asymptomatic individuals
c. It affects approximately 80 per cent of patients over the age of 80 years
d. It most commonly presents with bloody diarrhoea
e. Colonic resection and primary anastomosis is the management of choice

### 2. Consider complications of diverticular disease

a. Diverticular disease is the most common cause of colovesical fistula
b. They include adhesions
c. They include perforations
d. They include bowel obstruction
e. There is an increased risk of colorectal cancer

### 3. For the following scenarios choose the most appropriate complication of diverticular disease. Each option may be used once only

**Options**

A. Chronic pain
B. Colovesical fistula
C. Haemorrhage
D. Colovaginal fistula
E. Urinary tract infection
F. Coloileal fistula
G. Pericolic abscess
H. Acute diverticulitis
I. Bowel obstruction
J. Diverticulum perforation

1. A 60-year-old woman presents with lower abdominal pain and fever and on examination was found to have left iliac fossa tenderness that improves with IV antibiotics
2. An elderly woman with brown offensive vaginal discharge
3. A man with severe abdominal pain was found to have a profound hypotension, tachycardia and rigid abdomen with an absence of bowel sounds
4. A 72-year-old woman with left iliac fossa pain and swinging pyrexia. She was admitted and treated with IV antibiotics; however her symptoms did not resolve

### 4. What are the different clinical presentations of diverticular disease?

CRP, C-reactive protein; CT, computed tomography; FBC, full blood count; IV, intravenous

# EXPLANATION: DIVERTICULAR DISEASE

Diverticular disease is an acquired condition that primarily affects the **sigmoid colon** (can affect all parts of the large bowel except the rectum). In the Far East, right-sided diverticula are more common. A diverticulum is an outpouching of mucosa forced through the wall of the colon at sites of least resistance, i.e. sites of perforating arteries. It is a common condition that increases in prevalence with age. Approximately 50 per cent of those over 80 years have diverticula, but only 15–25 per cent are symptomatic. It is primarily caused by high intraluminal pressures as a result of hard stool associated with **low-fibre diets**.

Complications associated with diverticula include diverticulitis and pericolitis, a pericolic abscess, intraperitoneal perforation, haemorrhage, fistula formation, adhesions and bowel stricturing.

Clinical presentations include (4):
- **Chronic pain**: peridiverticular inflammation leads to a chronic recurrent left iliac fossa pain and chronic constipation, with small pellet-like faeces with episodic diarrhoea
- **Acute diverticulitis**: the patient presents with continuous severe left iliac fossa pain and systemic symptoms including a fever. There may be an associated localized peritonitis (presence of rebound tenderness or percussion tenderness and guarding)
- **Pericolic abscess**: presents similarly to acute diverticulitis but does not resolve with antibiotic therapy. If the abscess drains spontaneously there will be associated purulent diarrhoea
- **Diverticular perforation**: presents with an acute abdomen. There is severe abdominal pain and signs of peritonitis
- **Haemorrhage**: the patient passes fresh blood instead of stool. The bleeding usually stops spontaneously. Remember to exclude ischaemic colitis and colorectal cancer
- **Fistula formation**: the patient either presents with pneumaturia (colovesical fistula), purulent vaginal discharge (colovaginal fistula) or diarrhoea (coloileal fistula)
- **Obstruction**: is usually incomplete obstruction.

Patients should be investigated with blood analysis (FBC, renal profile, CRP, group and save), erect chest X-ray and abdominal X-ray. Gastrograffin enema with flexible sigmoidoscopy, CT scan or colonoscopy may also be indicated.

Management involves:
- High-fibre diet $\pm$ bran supplements
- Antispasmodics such as hyoscine or mebeverine if required
- For acute presentations IV cefuroxime and metronidazole should be commenced. The patient should also be nil by mouth and receive IV fluids
- In less severe cases of acute diverticulitis, the patient can be managed at home with oral cephalosporins and metronidazole
- Surgical management (usually a Hartmann's procedure) is indicated for the presence of a pericolic abscess, acute haemorrhage not managed conservatively, bowel perforation, fistulating disease and acute obstruction.

Answers
**1.** F T F F F
**2.** T T T T F
**3.** 1 – H, 2 – D, 3 – J, 4 – G
**4.** See explanation

## 5. Osmotic diarrhoea can be caused by

a. Crohn's disease
b. Hypercalcaemia
c. Hyperthyroidism
d. Magnesium sulphate
e. Villous adenoma

## 6. Regarding diarrhoea

a. Secretory diarrhoea resolves on fasting
b. Hypothyroidism causes dysmotility diarrhoea
c. Antibiotics are the mainstay of treatment
d. Anti-diarrhoeals should not be used early
e. *Clostridium difficile* is a common nosocomial infection treated with IV metronidazole or vancomycin

## 7. For the following scenarios choose the most appropriate diagnosis. Each option may be used once only

**Options**

A. Faecal impaction
B. Inflammatory bowel disease
C. *Escherichia coli* diarrhoea
D. Proton pump inhibitor use
E. Pseudomembranous colitis
F. Zollinger–Ellison syndrome
G. Phaeochromocytoma
H. Irritable bowel syndrome
I. Colorectal carcinoma
J. *Salmonella* sp. diarrhoea

1. A 40-year-old man with known peptic ulcer disease presents with diarrhoea. He is noted to have a high fasting blood gastrin level
2. A 20-year-old backpacker returns from a vacation in India and presents with an abrupt onset of watery diarrhoea that lasts for 3 days
3. A 70-year-old man with a history of colonic polyps presents with weight loss and change in bowel habit, and blood analysis reveals a microcytic anaemia
4. A 65-year-old patient recently treated for a chest infection one week ago develops fever, diarrhoea and crampy abdominal pain
5. A 22-year-old medical student has recurrent bouts of diarrhoea alternating with constipation, crampy abdominal pain eased on defaecation, and abdominal bloating

## 8. Write short notes on the different types of diarrhoea

CRP, C-reactive protein; ESR, erythrocyte sedimentation rate; FBC, full blood count; HIV, human immunodeficiency virus; IBD, inflammatory bowel disease; IV, intravenous; OGD, oesophago-gastroduodenoscopy; WHO, World Health Organization

# EXPLANATION: DIARRHOEA (I)

Diarrhoea is defined as defaecation of >300 g per day of loose stool. This definition is limited in clinical use and so the presence of reduced-consistency stool usually accompanied by increased frequency of defaecation is often used in practice to define diarrhoea.

Types and causes of diarrhoea are as follows (8):
- **Osmotic diarrhoea**: the presence of an osmotically active substance in the gut lumen leads to inhibition of water absorption. Causes include: disaccharidase deficiency, lactase deficiency, pancreatic insufficiency (chronic pancreatitis, cystic fibrosis), laxative abuse, bile salt malabsorption (Crohn's disease, ileal resection), viral gastroenteritis
- **Secretory diarrhoea**: active intestinal secretion of fluid and electrolytes as well as reduced absorption. Causes include: enterotoxins (*Vibrio cholerae, Escherichia coli*), inappropriate hormone secretion (gastrin, serotonin, glucagons, vasoactive intestinal peptide), stimulant laxatives, bile salt malabsorption, diabetic neuropathy, villous adenoma
- **Inflammatory diarrhoea**: disruption of the intestinal mucosa results in loss of fluid and blood, and defective electrolyte absorption. This occurs with infection: viral (rotavirus), bacterial, parasites (*Giardia lamblia, Cryptosporidium*). Ischaemia and inflammatory bowel disease (IBD) are other causes
- **Dysmotility diarrhoea** is seen in diabetic neuropathy, hyperthyroidism, phaeochromocytoma and irritable bowel syndrome
- **Other**: bowel malignancy, stool impaction, diverticular disease.

The differential diagnoses can be narrowed down with pertinent questions such as **characterization of stool** (colour, presence of blood or mucus, smell), **timing and relationship to meals** (osmotic diarrhoea ceases on fasting, while nocturnal diarrhoea and incontinence suggests an organic cause), **travel history, possible precipitants** such as eating out, **associated symptoms** (abdominal pain, vomiting, weight loss, fever), **relevant past medical history** (for example diabetes, HIV), **drug history** (recent antibiotic use, magnesium salts, $H_2$ antagonists) and **family history** (anyone else affected, IBD).

The examination may be unremarkable; however, there may be signs of dehydration. Examine for signs of systemic disease such as thyrotoxicosis. Abdominal examination may reveal surgical incision scars, abdominal tenderness, abdominal masses and the presence of blood on digital rectal examination.

Investigations should include stool microscopy, culture and sensitivity, blood analysis (FBC, renal profile, liver profile, ESR, CRP, amylase, thyroid profile, coeliac screen, tumour markers), abdominal X-ray, proctoscopy/sigmoidoscopy ± biopsy, barium enema, colonoscopy, OGD ± biopsy and duodenal aspirate.

The underlying cause should be treated. The patient should be rehydrated. Replacement oral rehydration solutions as recommended by the WHO can be used. **Avoid anti-diarrhoeal agents** (opioids and anticholinergics) as this may precipitate toxic megacolon.

---

Answers
**5.** T F F T F
**6.** F F F T F
**7.** 1 – F, 2 – C, 3 – I, 4 – E, 5 – H
**8.** See explanation

**9. Theme – Infective diarrhoea. For the following scenarios choose the most appropriate diagnosis. Each option may be used once only**

**Options**

A. *Clostridium perfringens* diarrhoea    F. *Shigella* sp. diarrhoea
B. *Campylobacter* sp. diarrhoea    G. Rotavirus
C. *Salmonella* sp. diarrhoea    H. *Clostridium difficile* diarrhoea
D. *Bacillus cereus* diarrhoea    I. *Staphylococcus aureus* diarrhoea
E. *Vibrio cholerae* diarrhoea    J. *Escherichia coli* diarrhoea

1. A 70-year-old woman was admitted with severe abdominal cramps and diarrhoea. She had recently been discharged from hospital following a presumed urinary tract infection
2. A 24-year-old man presents with diarrhoea following a recent holiday to the Far East. The diarrhoea lasts for 72 h
3. A 56-year-old man presents with ascending lower limb weakness following an episode of diarrhoea 4 weeks prior to the event. Choose the most likely cause of diarrhoea
4. A 4-year-old child develops cramping abdominal pain, fever, high-volume diarrhoea with frank blood. The incubation period was 48 h
5. A 19-year-old student develops vomiting and diarrhoea 24 h after ingestion of a left-over chicken sandwich

**10. The following conditions are associated with bloody diarrhoea**

a. *Vibrio cholerae* diarrhoea    d. Irritable bowel syndrome
b. *Escherichia coli* diarrhoea    e. Phaeochromocytoma
c. *Shigella* sp. diarrhoea

**11. A 25-year-old female lawyer presents with a 6-month history of poor sleep, left iliac fossa pain which is relieved by defaecation, intermittent diarrhoea and abdominal bloating. The GP has asked for advice**

a. What is the likely diagnosis?
b. What differential diagnosis would you consider in this patient?
c. What other information would you like from the history?
d. Create a management plan

CRP, C-reactive protein; GP, general practitioner; IBS, irritable bowel syndrome

## EXPLANATION: DIARRHOEA (II)

Specific infective causes of diarrhoea are shown below:

| Organism | Incubation period | Clinical features | Treatment |
|---|---|---|---|
| *Vibrio cholerae* | Hours to 6 days | Profuse watery diarrhoea with mucus flecks (rice-water diarrhoea), painless | Good hygiene measures, ciprofloxacin or tetracycline |
| *Escherichia coli* | 12–72 h | Watery diarrhoea ± haemorrhagic colitis (*E. coli 0157*), haemolytic uraemic syndrome | If systemic features are present use ciprofloxacin. In sepsis use gentamicin |
| *Salmonella* sp. | 12–48 h | Fever, abdominal pain, vomiting, diarrhoea | In severe cases use ciprofloxacin, erythromycin or co-trimoxazole |
| *Campylobacter* sp. | 48–96 h | Diarrhoea ± bloody diarrhoea, abdominal pain, Guillain–Barré syndrome, arthritis | In severe cases use ciprofloxacin, erythromycin or co-trimoxazole |
| *Shigella* sp. | 24–48 h | Diarrhoea containing blood and mucus, abdominal pain, fever | In severe cases use ciprofloxacin, erythromycin or co-trimoxazole |
| *Clostridium difficile* | Up to 4 weeks post antibiotic use | Ranges from mild diarrhoea to haemorrhagic colitis, abdominal pain | Discontinue other antibiotics, use oral metronidazole or vancomycin |

**Irritable bowel syndrome** (IBS) **(11a)** is a very common condition with **no recognizable organic cause**. The **Rome III criteria** for IBS state the presence of abdominal discomfort for 12 weeks, which need to be consecutive, of the previous year with two of the following features **(11c)**: relief on defaecation, onset associated with change in bowel frequency and onset associated with change in stool form.

Other symptoms include: >3 bowel movements/day *or* <3/week, abnormal stool form (hard or loose), abnormal stool passage (urgency/straining/tenesmus), mucus defaecation and bloating sensation.

A lot of patients with IBS do not fulfil the criteria above and most have less severe symptoms. **Stress worsens** or induces the **symptoms**. **Females** are more commonly affected. A typical history and unremarkable examination is usually sufficient for diagnosis. This is strengthened by a normal white cell count and CRP. **Warning features** that warrant further investigations include age >40 years at onset, persistent diarrhoea, nocturnal diarrhoea, weight loss, rectal bleeding and fever. One should consider and exclude other causes of diarrhoea, such as inflammatory bowel disease, infective diarrhoea and gastrointestinal malignancy **(11b)**, with a good history and investigations if necessary.

The patient should be **reassured**. Dietary measures including a **high-fibre diet** should be implemented. In some cases **psychotherapy** to reduce stress-related symptoms may be helpful. Patients with diarrhoea may benefit from **anti-diarrhoeals** such as loperamide. Those with constipation may benefit from **stool softeners and laxatives (11d)**.

Answers

**9.** 1 – H, 2 – J, 3 – B, 4 – F, 5 – C
**10.** F T T F F
**11.** See explanation

## 12. Regarding constipation

a. It is defined as the passage of hard stool with a reduction in frequency of defaecation
b. Loperamide may be indicated
c. Bulk laxatives are the first-line treatment
d. Stimulant laxatives may be indicated in complete constipation
e. Most patients do not require investigations

## 13. Causes of constipation include

a. Hypokalaemia
b. Hypocalcaemia
c. Magnesium salts

d. Diabetic neuropathy
e. Old age

## 14. For the following scenarios choose the most appropriate diagnosis. Each option may be used once only

**Options**

A. Porphyria
B. Faecal impaction
C. Diabetic neuropathy
D. Ferrous sulphate therapy
E. Diverticular disease

F. Mefenamic acid therapy
G. Rectal cancer
H. Immobility
I. Hypothyroidism
J. Cushing's syndrome

1. A 60-year-old man presents with weight loss, recent-onset constipation and tenesmus
2. A 29-year-old woman recently started on therapy for menorrhagia and anaemia visits her GP complaining of infrequent bowel motions and dark stools
3. A 42-year-old woman presents to her GP with weight gain, fatigue, cold intolerance and constipation
4. A 30-year-old woman who was recently started on the oral contraceptive pill develops abdominal pain, vomiting, constipation and is noted to have a polyneuropathy. On urinalysis it was noted that the urine changed colour on standing
5. A 72-year-old woman on an orthopaedic ward recovering from a hip replacement develops abdominal discomfort and constipation

CRP, C-reactive protein; FBC, full blood count; GP, general practitioner

## EXPLANATION: CONSTIPATION

Constipation is defined as the passage of less than 3 motions per week. However, in clinical practice, it is defined as a **reduction in frequency** compared to normal, associated with straining or discomfort on defaecation.

Causes of constipation include:
- **General**: dehydration, immobility, hypothyroidism, hypercalcaemia, porphyria, neuromuscular conditions such as Parkinson's disease, spinal nerve injury and diabetic neuropathy
- **Drugs**: opioids, anticholinergics (antidepressants, phenothiazines), aluminium salts and chronic laxative abuse
- **Gastrointestinal causes**: irritable bowel syndrome, intestinal obstruction, tumours, diverticular disease, congenital abnormalities such as Hirschsprung's disease, anal fissures and perianal abscesses.

Pertinent questions in the history include:
- Duration of constipation
- Is it recurrent?
- Characterization of stool (form, colour, presence of blood or mucus)
- History of incontinence
- Associated symptoms such as alternating diarrhoea, abdominal pain, vomiting, weight loss, anorexia
- Psychological background
- Past medical history
- Drug history
- Family history of colorectal cancer.

Examination should involve an abdominal and digital rectal examination. Proctoscopy may be helpful. **Most patients do not warrant investigations**. In the presence of persistent constipation or associated warning symptoms, blood analysis (FBC, renal profile, liver profile, thyroid profile, calcium profile, CRP), stool culture, abdominal X-ray, barium enema with sigmoidoscopy, or colonoscopy should be considered.

Management options are:
- Lifestyle advice including increased fluid and fibre intake
- Treat the underlying cause
- Laxatives:
  - **bulk-forming laxatives** (ispaghula, methylcellulose): soften the stool and increase bowel frequency through increased faecal mass and water content
  - **stool softeners** (docusate sodium, arachis oil)
  - **osmotic laxatives** (lactulose, movicol, phosphate enema): increase water in the large-bowel lumen by reducing absorption and increasing secretion
  - **stimulant laxatives** (senna, bisacodyl): increase intestinal motility and alter electrolyte transport by the intestinal mucosa. These should be avoided in obstruction.

Answers
**12.** T F F F T
**13.** T F F T F
**14.** 1 – G, 2 – D, 3 – I, 4 – A, 5 – H

## 15. Regarding colorectal cancer

a. Calcium is a risk factor for colorectal cancer
b. Tubular adenoma have a higher risk of malignant transformation than villous adenoma
c. Obstruction is more common in right-sided lesions than left-sided lesions
d. About 45 per cent of tumours are found in the rectum
e. About 5 per cent present with bowel perforation

## 16. Consider familial cases of colorectal cancer

a. Familial adenomatous polyposis (FAP) is an autosomal recessive condition
b. FAP accounts for 10 per cent of all colorectal cancers
c. Parathyroid adenomas are an extra-colonic feature of Gardner's syndrome
d. Hereditary non-polyposis colon cancers (HNPCC) are often left sided
e. Endometrial cancer is associated with HNPCC

## 17. A 22-year-old man whose father died of colorectal cancer at a young age presents with change in bowel habit and rectal bleeding. Colonoscopy revealed hundreds of polyps in the colon

a. What is the likely diagnosis?
b. What is the associated syndrome?
c. What are possible extracolonic features associated with this condition?
d. What is the surveillance protocol for first-degree relatives?

## 18. Write short notes on hereditary non-polyposis colon cancer

FAP, familial adenomatous polyposis; HNPCC, hereditary non-polyposis colon cancer

# EXPLANATION: COLORECTAL CANCER (I)

Colorectal cancer is the second commonest cause of cancer deaths (11 per cent) in the Western world. It affects men and women equally, but rectal cancer has a slight preponderance in males. The peak incidence occurs in the seventh decade. Seventy-five per cent of cases are sporadic.

Risk factors for colorectal cancer include:
- **Age**: increased incidence with age
- **Diet**: rich in red meat and animal fat increases the risk. Folate and calcium are protective
- **Polyps** (adenoma–carcinoma sequence): adenomatous polyps increase the risk of adenocarcinoma. Association with malignancy depends on size, degree of dysplasia and histology. There are three types:
  - tubular adenoma (80 per cent): <5 per cent are malignant
  - tubulovillous adenoma (13 per cent): 20 per cent are malignant
  - villous adenoma (7 per cent): 35–40 per cent are malignant
- **Hereditary syndromes**:
  - **familial adenomatous polyposis (FAP)**: an autosomal dominant condition with a point mutation in the adenomatous polyposis coli tumour suppressor gene on chromosome 5q21. Twenty-five per cent are new mutations. It accounts for about 2 per cent of colorectal cancers. Symptoms usually manifest from age 16–40 years. Cancer develops in 100 per cent by age 60 years if untreated **(17a)**. Family members should be screened from the age of 12 years to 35 years, either annually or every two years, with flexible sigmoidoscopy. After 35 years screening should be three-yearly. Genetic testing is also available **(17d)**
  - **Gardner's syndrome (17b)**: a variant of FAP with extracolonic features such as periampullary lesions, gastric polyps, dermoids, Turcot syndrome, hypertrophy of retinal pigment epithelium, mandible osteomata, thyroid cancer, epidermoid and subcutaneous cysts **(17c)**
- **Hereditary non-polyposis colon cancer (HNPCC) (18)**: is an autosomal dominant condition, with germline mutations in one of six mismatch repair genes being the underlying genetic defect in most kindreds. It accounts for 1–5 per cent of colorectal cancers. The cancer tends to be right sided and occurs on average at age 45 years. There are two types: Lynch I which is isolated colorectal cancer and Lynch II which is associated with small bowel, ovarian or endometrial cancer
- **Inflammatory bowel disease** (higher risk with ulcerative colitis)
- **Smoking**
- **Past medical history of colorectal carcinoma**
- **Positive family history**.

Answers
**15.** F F F T T
**16.** F F F F T
**17.** See explanation
**18.** See explanation

### 19. Consider colorectal cancer

a. Right-sided lesions tend to be morphologically exophytic
b. The commonest site for colon cancer is the descending colon
c. Dukes' B disease is associated with a 60 per cent 5-year survival
d. CA-125 may be diagnostic
e. Faecal occult blood testing is a diagnostic tool

### 20. Consider management of colorectal cancer

a. A right hemicolectomy involves resection of the distal ileum
b. Tumours in the splenic flexure are resected using the extended left hemicolectomy approach
c. An abdominoperineal resection is reserved for tumours that are <10 cm from the anal verge
d. Colon cancer is sensitive to radiotherapy
e. Surgery is the only curative option

### 21. Outline the management options for colorectal carcinoma

---

CEA, carcinoembryonic antigen; CT, computed tomography; FBC, full blood count; PET, positron emission tomography; TNM, tumour, node, metastasis

## EXPLANATION: COLORECTAL CANCER (II)

More than 90 per cent of colorectal cancers are adenocarcinomas. They are grossly described as ulcerative (most common), exophytic or polypoid (usually right-sided tumours), annular and submucosal infiltrative. Sites of colorectal cancer are shown below (right):

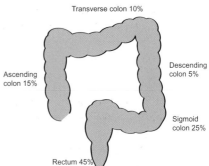

Staging uses the TNM (tumour, node, metastasis) classification:
- Tis: carcinoma *in situ*
- T1: invades the submucosa
- T2: invades the muscularis propria
- T3: invades into the subserosa or nonperitonized pericolic tissue
- T4: invades other organs or perforates the visceral peritoneum
- N1: 1–3 regional nodes affected
- N2: ≥4 regional nodes affected
- M: distant metastases

| Stage | | Dukes' classification | 5-year survival |
|---|---|---|---|
| Stage 0 | Tis N0 M0 | | |
| Stage I | T1/2 N0 M0 | Dukes' A | 80–90% |
| Stage II | T3/4 N0 M0 | Dukes' B | 60% |
| Stage III | Any T, N1/2, M0 | Dukes' C | 30% |
| Stage IV | Any T, any N, M1 | Dukes' D | <5% |

Colorectal cancer spreads either locally to adjacent viscera, via lymphatics to lymph nodes, via the bloodstream to the liver, lungs and bone, as well as by transcoelomic spread.

Patients with left-sided lesions present with **bowel obstruction** in 15–25 per cent of cases, **bowel perforation** in 5–8 per cent of cases, **change in bowel habit, rectal bleeding, tenesmus, weight loss and anorexia**. Right-sided lesions are associated with weight loss, anorexia, symptoms of anaemia (tiredness, shortness of breath, chest pain) and history of diarrhoea. Useful investigations include blood analysis (FBC, renal profile, liver profile, coagulation profile, group and save, CEA, CA19–9), faecal occult blood testing for screening, colonoscopy and biopsy, chest X-ray, CT scan (chest, abdomen and pelvis) for staging, and a PET scan.

Management options are **(21)**:
- **Surgical therapy**: *Right hemicolectomy* for right-sided tumours. The distal ileum is resected up to the transverse colon proximal to the middle colic artery. *Extended right hemicolectomy* for transverse colon tumours. Resection as for right hemicolectomy but includes the whole of the transverse colon. *Left hemicolectomy* for left-sided tumours. Segmental resection of transverse colon distal to the middle colic artery up to the rectum. *Low anterior resection* for tumours 4–5 cm from the anal verge. The distal descending colon is removed up to the upper two-thirds of the rectum. *Abdominoperineal resection* for tumours <5 cm from the anal verge. This requires removal of the anus and a colostomy
- **Adjuvant therapy** in the form of chemotherapy, or combined with radiotherapy for rectal cancers
- **Palliative care** including palliative resection or bypass, stenting and symptom control.

Answers
**19.** T F T F F
**20.** T F F F T
**21.** See explanation

## 22. Consider the anatomy of the anal canal

a. The anal canal extends from the anal verge to the levator ani muscles
b. The anal canal mucosa changes at the dentate line
c. The distal anal canal is lined by columnar epithelium and is sensitive to pain
d. Haemorrhoids occur in the 3, 6 and 9 o'clock positions as viewed in the lithotomy position
e. The levator ani makes up the external sphincter component

## 23. Regarding haemorrhoids

a. They can present with faecal incontinence
b. Portal hypertension is a risk factor
c. They are usually painful
d. Second-degree haemorrhoids require digital manipulation for reduction
e. For strangulated haemorrhoids the initial management is conservative

## 24. Causes of pruritus ani include

a. Diabetes
b. Hypertension
c. Skin melanoma
d. Anal fissure
e. *Enterobius* infection

## EXPLANATION: ANAL AND PERIANAL DISORDERS (I)

The anal canal is about 4 cm long, extending from the anal verge to the levator ani muscles. From the anal verge to the dentate line it is lined by stratified squamous epithelium; above this point the epithelium is columnar. The upper verge of the anal canal is thrown into mucosal folds (columns of Morgagni) each containing a branch of the superior rectal artery and vein. The figure below gives a summary of anal canal anatomy:

**Haemorrhoids (piles)** are enlarged and engorged anal cushions that can bleed, prolapse or result in mucus or faecal incontinence during the passage of flatus. Fifty per cent of the population is affected. They are classified into **(25a)**:

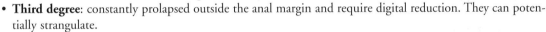

Columnar epithelium
Pelvic and abdominal lymph node drainage

Squamous epithelium
Inguinal lymph node drainage

Levator ani
Dentate line
Internal sphincter
External sphincter mechanism (puborectalis sling)

- **First degree**: never prolapse out of the anal canal
- **Second degree**: prolapse out of the anus on defaecation and reduce spontaneously
- **Third degree**: constantly prolapsed outside the anal margin and require digital reduction. They can potentially strangulate.

Haemorrhoids are believed to arise from increased straining secondary to constipation and impaired venous return, for example in pregnancy, portal hypertension, abdominal or pelvic tumours **(25b)**.

They often produce intermittent symptoms that last for a few days to weeks. **Constipation** is a precipitating factor. Patients often note **fresh blood** on toilet paper or on the surface of stool, or sprayed inside the toilet bowl. Some present with pruritus ani (see box below for causes of pruritus ani), mucus or faecal incontinence on passing flatus, or a perianal lump. Occasionally, patients present acutely with pain if the haemorrhoid is thrombosed or strangulated.

> **Causes of pruritis ani**
> - Poor hygiene
> - Anal fissure
> - *Enterobius* and *Candida* infection
> - Anorectal carcinoma
> - Bowen's disease
> - Jaundice
> - Haemorrhoids
> - Anal fistula
> - Crohn's disease
> - Skin melanoma
> - Diabetes

Continued on page 133

Answers

25. **A 68-year-old man with constipation presents with fresh rectal bleeding on defaecation. There is no history of weight loss. The blood stains the bowl and is not mixed in with the stool. At proctoscopy haemorrhoids were noted**

   a. How are haemorrhoids classified?
   b. How do haemorrhoids arise?
   c. What are the management options available?
   d. What important differential diagnoses should you consider in a patient who presents with rectal bleeding?

## EXPLANATION: ANAL AND PERIANAL DISORDERS (I)  Cont'd from page 131

An abdominal examination is essential to exclude masses. A digital rectal examination may reveal prolapsed haemorrhoids and external skin tags (a sign of longstanding haemorrhoids). Note on internal examination haemorrhoids are not palpable. During withdrawal of a proctoscope, haemorrhoids may be noted in the classical positions (3, 7 and 11 o'clock in the lithotomy position):

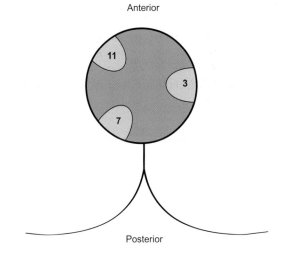

It is important to consider colorectal carcinoma as the underlying cause of rectal bleeding despite the presence of haemorrhoids **(25d)**.

Management of haemorrhoids should include **(25c)**:

- General measures such as a high-fibre diet, reduce straining on defaecation, heeding the call of defaecation and good anal hygiene should be advised
- Medical management with the use of topical agents and laxatives
- Interventional options are:
  - **injection sclerotherapy** (first degree): 5 per cent phenol injected submucosally at the pedicles of the haemorrhoids as an outpatient procedure
  - **Barron's banding** (second degree): rubber band ligation of the neck of the haemorrhoid as an outpatient procedure to obliterate vessels
  - **cryotherapy**
  - **infrared therapy**
  - **haemorrhoidectomy** (third degree): laxatives are required pre- and post-operatively. It is a very painful procedure.

For thrombosed or strangulated haemorrhoids, the initial management is conservative with analgesia, stool softeners, ice packs, elevation of the foot of the bed and then the haemorrhoids can be either injected or surgically excised.

Answers

**25.** See explanation (pages 131 and 133)

## 26. Regarding perianal pathology

    **a.** A sentinel pile is associated with haemorrhoids
    **b.** Psoriasis is a known cause of anal fissures
    **c.** Anal fissures are more common in men
    **d.** Anal fissures usually present in the midline
    **e.** Diltiazem is a therapeutic option for anal fissures

## 27. Regarding anal fistulae

    **a.** They can be associated with perianal sepsis
    **b.** They do not cross the anal sphincter
    **c.** Crohn's disease classically present with multiple fistulae
    **d.** Patients classically present with rectal bleeding
    **e.** Surgical management of low fistulae involves the use of a seton suture

## 28. What is Goodsall's rule?

# EXPLANATION: ANAL AND PERIANAL DISORDERS (II)

## ANAL FISSURE

An anal fissure is a linear tear in the anal epithelium below the dentate line. It is usually present in the midline; posterior tears are more common, while anterior ones are associated with the postpartum period. They are more common in women. They usually occur after the passage of hard stool. Other causes include Crohn's disease, anal cancer, psoriasis, TB, syphilis and trauma.

Patients present with **severe pain during defaecation**, described as broken glass or stabbing pain. The discomfort lasts for several hours due to sphincter spasm. Patients often have associated fresh rectal bleeding on defaecation. On examination, a sentinel pile (small skin tag) may be present at the superficial end of the fissure. The fissure is usually concealed by sphincter spasm. Internal examination is usually excruciating and unnecessary. The diagnosis is largely based on the history. Management is as follows:

- **Dietary advice**
- **Conservative**: glyceryl trinitrate 0.2 per cent ointment is helpful in 60 per cent of cases. Concentrations can be increased. Warn the patients that headaches are a common side-effect. An alternative is diltiazem cream. Stool softeners and laxatives can also be prescribed
- **Surgery**: lateral internal sphincterostomy performed under general anaesthetic. Lord's procedure or anal stretch is best avoided.

## ANAL FISTULA

A fistula is an abnormal track between two epithelial surfaces; in this case the anorectal epithelium and skin. They are associated with previous perianal sepsis, Crohn's disease, anorectal carcinoma, TB, radiotherapy and immunosuppression.

Anal fistulae are classified as: **low anal fistulae** (do not cross the anal sphincter muscle) and **high anal fistulae** (cross the anal sphincter).

The track of fistulae can be predicted with Goodsall's rule **(28)**: 'if the external opening of a fistula is behind a line drawn transversely across the anus (see figure opposite), the internal opening of the fistula is single and in the midline. If the external opening is in front of the line, the track opens radially into the anal canal.' Horseshoe fistulae confound this rule.

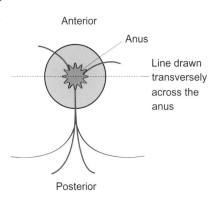

Patients often present with intermittent discharge of faecal-stained mucus around the perianal region, and perianal irritation. This condition should be investigated with a colonoscopy. Complex fistulae should be imaged with an MRI scan. Low fistulae are allowed to heal by granulation after exploration and laying open of the tract (fistulotomy) under general anaesthetic. For high fistulae, surgery is more complex, often involving the use of a seton suture placed along the fistula, and later a flap technique conserving the sphincter.

Answers
**26.** F T F T T
**27.** T F T F F
**28.** See explanation

## 29. Regarding perianal conditions

**a.** Perianal haematomas when painful are best treated with antibiotics
**b.** Ischiorectal abscesses are the most common type of anorectal abscesses
**c.** Ulcerative colitis is a common cause of anorectal abscesses
**d.** Anorectal abscesses are usually situated above the levator ani
**e.** Anorectal abscess may be a presenting feature of anorectal cancer

## 30. Which of the following are true?

**a.** Rectal prolapse is most common in the extremes of age
**b.** Rectal prolapse tends to occur in multiparous women
**c.** Pilonidal sinus is more common in females
**d.** Pilonidal sinus is best treated with excision and closure
**e.** Pilonidal sinus is more common in obese individuals

TB, tuberculosis

## EXPLANATION: ANAL AND PERIANAL DISORDERS (III)

**A perianal haematoma** is a **subcutaneous collection of blood in the perianal region** due to the passage of hard stool. It presents with acute perianal pain worsened by movement or defaecation. On examination, a small (approximately 4 mm) dark-blue berry-shaped mass is visible at the anal margin. It is treated conservatively or by incision and drainage under local anaesthetic.

An **anorectal abscess** usually begins as an acute purulent infection of the anal glands following obstruction of the gland ducts. The glands lie between the internal and external sphincters. The abscesses can be classified as:
• **Perianal**: about 45 per cent of cases
• **Ischiorectal**: about 30 per cent of cases
• **Intersphincteric**: about 20 per cent of cases
• **Supralevator**: about 5 per cent of cases.

Patients usually present with throbbing anal pain, which is worse on sitting and defaecation. Occasionally they may have a purulent per rectal discharge. They often have systemic symptoms and signs of infection. A mass or cellulitic area may be visible in the perianal region. Digital rectal examination may reveal a fluctuant tender mass. It is important to exclude diabetes mellitus, Crohn's disease, anorectal carcinoma and TB. If the infection is caught in an early phase, antibiotics may be sufficient. Otherwise surgical incision and drainage is required. The wound is packed with daily dressings and left to heal by secondary intention.

**A rectal prolapse** is a **protrusion of the rectal tissue via the anal canal**. It is either **partial** (mucosal prolapse) or **complete** (muscle wall and mucosal protrusion). The former is more common in children. Prolapses are more common in women with a poor gynaecological and obstetric history.

Patients often present with a mass arising from the rectum, soiling of underwear and possible rectal bleeding. On examination, the prolapse may be visible, and may have areas of ulceration. There may be associated uterovaginal prolapse. Sigmoidoscopy should be performed.

Management involves pelvic floor exercises and stool softeners in the first instance. Some cases require surgical therapy. A small partial prolapse can be band ligated or treated with injection sclerotherapy. Other forms require an abdominal approach (rectopexy) or perineal approach (Delorme's procedure).

**Pilonidal sinus (nest of hairs)** is trapping of hair in the natal cleft and leads to the formation of pits with hair debris causing a chronic subcutaneous infection. It affects males more often than females (ratio of 4:1), and is more common in obese and hairy people, and those from the Mediterranean, Middle East and Asia.

Patients present with a painful natal cleft with clear or purulent discharge. There may be an abscess or recurrent subcutaneous infections. Hair from the natal cleft should be removed. Antibiotics may be sufficient for an early infection. Abscesses should be incised and drained, while a chronic sinus should be laid open or excised with packing.

Continued on page 139

Answers
**29.** F F F F T
**30.** T T F F T

### 31. Anal cancer

a. Is radiosensitive
b. Is usually treated surgically
c. Is associated with human papilloma virus
d. The most common type is adenocarcinoma
e. Can spread to the inguinal nodes

### 32. Choose the most appropriate diagnosis for the case scenarios below. Each option may only be used once

**Options**

A. Second-degree haemorrhoids
B. Anal cancer
C. Perianal abscess
D. Third-degree haemorrhoids
E. Anal fissure
F. Anal fistula
G. Perianal haematoma
H. Pruritus ani
I. Pilonidal sinus

1. A 50-year-old man presents with excruciating pain on defaecation. On examination a sentinel pile is noted, and digital rectal examination is not possible due to sphincter spasm
2. A 42-year-old long-distance lorry driver presents with a lump and pain in the natal cleft. Inspection reveals a discharging raised area
3. A 34-year-old patient with diabetes presents with a perianal tender mass and yellow discharge per rectum. On examination she is pyrexial with erythematosus perianal skin, and a fluctuant mass is noted
4. A 70-year-old hypothyroid woman presents with a 3-day history of painless fresh rectal bleeding that is present on wiping herself and is occasionally sprayed over the toilet bowl. On examination a plum-sized mass is seen protruding from the anal canal. The mass is reducible

## EXPLANATION: ANAL AND PERIANAL DISORDERS (III) Cont'd from page 137

### ANAL CARCINOMA

Anal carcinoma is a rare neoplasm. More than 80 per cent are squamous cell carcinomas. Other tumours include adenocarcinomas, lymphomas and melanomas.

Those below the dentate line are often well differentiated and have a better prognosis. They are more common in men and spread to the inguinal nodes. Tumours above the dentate line are usually poorly differentiated and more common in women. They spread to the pelvic lymph nodes.

There is an increased incidence in sexually active homosexual men, cigarette smokers and human papilloma virus infection.

Most patients present with perianal pain and rectal bleeding. Sphincter involvement leads to faecal incontinence. A quarter of patients have a palpable mass on examination. Advanced cases can present with fistulae and palpable inguinal nodes.

Anal carcinoma is treated with chemotherapy and radiotherapy. Surgical resection is indicated for small tumours without sphincter involvement, tumours that do not respond to radiotherapy, and large tumours that cause obstruction.

Answers
**31.** T F T F T
**32.** 1 – E, 2 – I, 3 – C, 4 – D

33. List the medical and surgical differential diagnoses of a patient presenting with right upper quadrant pain

34. Regarding an acute abdomen

     **a.** Sudden onset of pain suggests inflammation
     **b.** Absence of bowel sounds suggests bowel obstruction
     **c.** Strong analgesia should be avoided until a differential diagnosis is achieved
     **d.** It is advisable to start broad-spectrum antibiotics
     **e.** It is important to rule out diabetes mellitus

# EXPLANATION: ACUTE ABDOMEN (I)

The hallmark of an acute abdomen is sudden onset of severe pain centred around the abdomen. The common causes of an acute abdomen are summarized in the figure below **(33) (36d)**:

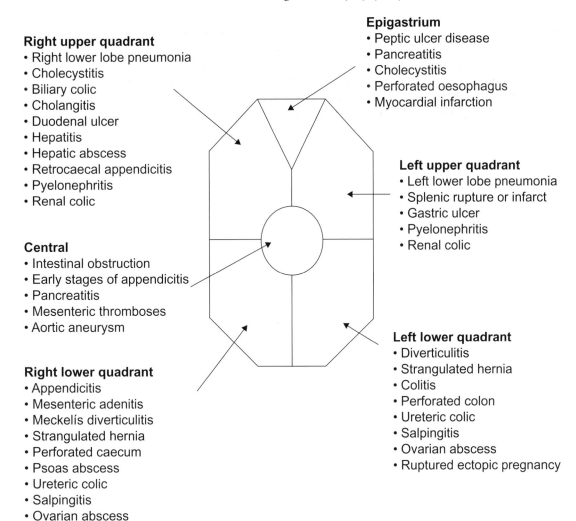

**Right upper quadrant**
• Right lower lobe pneumonia
• Cholecystitis
• Biliary colic
• Cholangitis
• Duodenal ulcer
• Hepatitis
• Hepatic abscess
• Retrocaecal appendicitis
• Pyelonephritis
• Renal colic

**Central**
• Intestinal obstruction
• Early stages of appendicitis
• Pancreatitis
• Mesenteric thromboses
• Aortic aneurysm

**Right lower quadrant**
• Appendicitis
• Mesenteric adenitis
• Meckelís diverticulitis
• Strangulated hernia
• Perforated caecum
• Psoas abscess
• Ureteric colic
• Salpingitis
• Ovarian abscess
• Ruptured ectopic pregnancy

**Epigastrium**
• Peptic ulcer disease
• Pancreatitis
• Cholecystitis
• Perforated oesophagus
• Myocardial infarction

**Left upper quadrant**
• Left lower lobe pneumonia
• Splenic rupture or infarct
• Gastric ulcer
• Pyelonephritis
• Renal colic

**Left lower quadrant**
• Diverticulitis
• Strangulated hernia
• Colitis
• Perforated colon
• Ureteric colic
• Salpingitis
• Ovarian abscess
• Ruptured ectopic pregnancy

Continued on page 143

Answers

**33.** See explanation
**34.** F F F F T

35. **For the following scenarios choose the most appropriate diagnosis. Each option may be used once only**

### Options

| | |
|---|---|
| **A.** Acute pancreatitis | **F.** Ischaemic colitis |
| **B.** Abdominal aortic aneurysm | **G.** Small-bowel obstruction secondary to intussusception |
| **C.** Splenic rupture | **H.** Small-bowel obstruction secondary to adhesions |
| **D.** Strangulated femoral hernia | **I.** Perforated peptic ulcer |
| **E.** Irreducible femoral hernia | **J.** Acute cholecystitis |

1. A 70-year-old woman with atrial fibrillation presents with central abdominal pain and rectal bleeding
2. A 49-year-old man on regular analgesia for rheumatoid arthritis presents with hypotension and tachycardia, as well as a rigid and silent abdomen
3. A 60-year-old woman presents with a painful hot red lump below and lateral to the pubic tubercle
4. A 21-year-old man presents with upper abdominal pain and bilious vomiting. On examination a Lanz incision is noted. He has generalized tenderness and hyperactive bowel sounds
5. A 40-year-old man with known history of gallstones presents with severe epigastric pain radiating to the back

36. **A 54-year-old woman with a history of rheumatoid arthritis presents with severe epigastric pain and collapse. On examination her blood pressure was 80/42 mmHg and she had a rigid abdomen with diminished bowel sounds**

a. Outline the immediate management of this patient
b. What investigations would you perform?
c. What is the most likely diagnosis?
d. What other differential diagnoses should be considered?

CRP, C-reactive protein; CT, computed tomography; ECG, electrocardiogram; FBC, full blood count

## EXPLANATION: ACUTE ABDOMEN (I)  Cont'd from page 141

Distinct features in the history can help identify potential causes of an acute abdomen. The **age** of the patient can differentiate the differential diagnosis, for example mesenteric adenitis is common in children, and diverticulitis is more common in the elderly. The **site of the pain** as illustrated on page 141 can guide the clinician. **Sudden onset** suggests pathology such as perforation, while **gradual onset** often suggests inflammation. Furthermore, **colicky pain** implies viscus obstruction, while **constant pain** suggests inflammation or ischaemia. Exacerbation with movement makes peritoneal inflammation more likely. In females a menstrual history should be elicited.

Examination of the patient should entail a general examination for signs of shock, abdominal examination, external genitalia examination and a digital rectal examination.

Patients should only be investigated **(36b)** after resuscitation, with blood analysis (FBC, renal profile, liver profile, coagulation profile, glucose, amylase, CRP, group and save, blood cultures), urinalysis, a pregnancy test, an arterial blood gas, ECG, erect chest X-ray (subdiaphragmatic gas indicates bowel perforation), abdominal X-ray, CT scan if needed and laparoscopy ± laparotomy.

Management **(36a)** includes resuscitation using the ABC approach, insertion of a urinary catheter to monitor urine output, and placing the patient nil by mouth. Opioid analgesia is often required and broad-spectrum antibiotics may be indicated. Surgery may be required depending on the cause or if conservative management fails.

Answers

**35.** 1 – F, 2 – I, 3 – D, 4 – H, 5 – A
**36.** a and b – see explanation (page 143), c – the diagnosis is perforated peptic ulcer, d – see explanation (page 141)

**37. Consider acute appendicitis**

    **a.** It is the most common surgical emergency
    **b.** It characteristically commences with right iliac fossa pain
    **c.** Vomiting is a key feature
    **d.** Most cases present with urinary frequency
    **e.** Tenderness is localized to McBurney's point (a third of the way along a line drawn from the umbilicus to the anterior superior iliac spine)

**38. Describe the anatomy of McBurney's point**

# EXPLANATION: ACUTE ABDOMEN (II)

**Acute appendicitis** is the most common surgical emergency in the developed world, and it is characterized by inflammation of the vermiform appendix. The majority of patients are between the age of 10 and 30 years. The average lifetime incidence is 6 per cent. Appendicitis occurs when the lumen of the appendix is obstructed by a faecolith, foreign body, lymphoid follicle, caecal tumour or a carcinoid tumour.

Patients present with abdominal pain that classically starts as a central **colicky umbilical pain, and then migrates to localize in the right iliac fossa**. Patients are often anorexic with nausea and occasional vomiting. Patients with a pelvic appendix often have diarrhoea and urinary frequency.

Signs are:
- Mild pyrexia, tachycardia
- Fetor oris, facial flushing, tongue furring
- Patient lies still
- Right hip may be flexed due to psoas muscle irritation
- Abdominal examination reveals:
  - tenderness over the right iliac fossa (**McBurney's point (38)** – two-thirds of the way along a line drawn from the umbilicus to the anterior superior iliac spine) $\pm$ guarding
  - the presence of percussion tenderness
  - Rovsing's sign may be positive: pressure over the left iliac fossa on palpation produces pain in the right iliac fossa
- Digital rectal examination may be painful with a low-lying appendix.

The natural course of appendicitis can be resolution, formation of an appendix mass (omentum and small bowel adhere to the appendix), an appendix abscess (in association with a mass there is swinging pyrexia), or appendix perforation.

Acute appendicitis is managed with open or laparoscopic appendicectomy with perioperative antibiotics. An appendix mass is often initially managed conservatively with IV fluids and antibiotics, with a close monitoring of the mass size. If symptoms resolve, elective appendicectomy is performed in a few months, otherwise an urgent appendicectomy is performed. If there are signs of an abscess (swinging fever, tachycardia, increasing mass size) then the abscess should be drained via an incision lateral to McBurney's point. Following resolution an appendicectomy should be performed.

Continued on page 147

Answers

**37.** T F F F F
**38.** See explanation

**39. Regarding small-bowel obstruction**

    **a.** Adhesions are the most common cause

    **b.** Constipation is an early feature

    **c.** Small-bowel volvulus can lead to strangulation

    **d.** Abdominal X-rays show distended loops of bowel in the periphery

    **e.** Surgical intervention is the first line of management

**40. Regarding large-bowel obstruction**

    **a.** Diverticulitis is the commonest cause

    **b.** Vomiting is an early feature

    **c.** Caecal perforation is a risk in the presence of a competent ileocaecal valve

    **d.** Ogilvie's syndrome is a complication of electrolyte imbalance

    **e.** A flatus tube can help manage a caecal volvulus

IV, intravenous; TB, tuberculosis

## EXPLANATION: ACUTE ABDOMEN (II) Cont'd from page 145

The causes of **bowel obstruction** can be mechanical or functional. The functional causes (ileus or **Ogilvie's syndrome**) are either in the post-operative period, due to metabolic causes such as diabetes mellitus, electrolyte disturbance and as a consequence of drugs (opiates, antidepressants), intra-abdominal sepsis and trauma. Mechanical causes of obstruction can be classified as:

|  | **Small bowel** | **Large bowel** |
| --- | --- | --- |
| Luminal | Food bolus<br>Foreign body<br>Gallstone ileus | Faecal impaction |
| Intramural | Strictures: Crohn's disease<br>Neoplasm<br>Ischaemic<br>Intussusception<br>Infective causes: TB | Carcinoma (commonest cause)<br>Strictures: diverticulitis, ischaemic<br>Hirschsprung's disease |
| Extramural | Adhesions (commonest cause)<br>Herniae<br>Volvulus<br>Gross lymphadenopathy | Volvulus<br>Diverticular abscess<br>Gross lymphadenopathy |

**Small-bowel obstruction** presents with **generalized colicky abdominal pain centred over the upper abdomen.** Vomiting usually follows the pain. Bilous vomiting indicates a higher level of obstruction, and faeculant vomiting suggests lower levels of obstruction. Progressive abdominal distension occurs, but **constipation is a late feature**. The presence of scars suggests adhesions. A distended tympanic abdomen may be noted, and in thin individuals visible peristalsis is present. High-pitched tinkling bowel sounds are audible. Hernia orifices should be checked for overlying skin changes, tenderness and irreducible masses.

In **large-bowel obstruction**, the patient often presents with **generalized constant abdominal pain centred over the lower abdomen**. Vomiting occurs late, while absolute **constipation is an early feature**. Abdominal distension is also noted. Tenderness over the right iliac fossa (caecum) suggests impending perforation. Caecal perforation is possible in the presence of a competent ileocaecal valve.

Abdominal X-ray plays an important role in diagnosis. Small-bowel obstruction presents with central gas shadows and valvulae conniventes (visible lines going all the way across the small bowel), while X-rays of large-bowel obstruction show a peripheral pattern of gas shadows, absence of gas in the rectum and haustral patterns. Gastrograffin swallow or enema can help demarcate the level of obstruction. Patients should be resuscitated and be placed nil by mouth. IV fluids are administered. A nasogastric tube should be inserted on free-flow drainage. Any electrolyte abnormalities should be corrected. The underlying cause should be treated, for example insertion of a flatus tube or a flexible sigmoidoscope may be therapeutic for a sigmoid volvulus. Surgical indications are strangulation, peritonitis, closed loop obstruction (i.e. the bowel is obstructed at two points) and when conservative measures fail.

Answers
**39.** T F T F F
**40.** F F T T F

### 41. Regarding abdominal hernias

**a.** Strangulated hernias are a surgical emergency
**b.** A Richter's hernia presents with signs of obstruction
**c.** Malnutrition is a risk factor for acquired abdominal hernias
**d.** Chronic prostatic symptoms predispose to abdominal hernias
**e.** Incarcerated hernias are often reducible

### 42. Regarding inguinal hernias

**a.** Direct hernias are usually congenital
**b.** Direct hernias are more common than indirect hernias
**c.** Indirect inguinal hernias are more likely to strangulate than direct hernias
**d.** At surgery, indirect inguinal hernias are medial to the inferior epigastric vessels
**e.** Direct inguinal hernias often descend into the scrotum

### 43. Consider femoral hernias

**a.** They are more common in males
**b.** They account for 30 per cent of all abdominal hernias
**c.** They have a high risk of strangulation
**d.** The neck of the hernia lies below and medial to the pubic tubercle
**e.** They can be managed conservatively

### 44. Draw the anatomy of the inguinal canal

COPD, chronic obstructive pulmonary disease

## EXPLANATION: ACUTE ABDOMEN (III)

A hernia is the **abnormal protrusion of an organ or part of an organ through a defect in the wall of its containing cavity**. Abdominal hernias occur at sites of abdominal wall weakness. The weakness can be:
- **Congenital**: for example a patent processus vaginalis leading to an indirect inguinal hernia, or failure of closure of the umbilical orifice leading to an umbilical hernia
- **Acquired**: primary (develop at natural weak points) or secondary (develop at sites of injury).

Factors that predispose to acquired hernias include:
- Increased abdominal pressure: heavy lifting, chronic cough (for example in COPD), straining to pass urine or defaecate, and abdominal distension (for example ascites)
- Weakened abdominal wall: increased age, surgical incision, collagen disorders, malnutrition and paralysis of motor nerves.

Hernias are often described as:
- **Reducible**: the contents of the hernia can be returned to its original cavity by gentle manipulation
- **Irreducible/incarcerated**: the contents of the hernia cannot be returned to its original cavity, for example the abdominal cavity due to adhesions
- **Strangulated**: the blood supply to the hernia contents is compromised and hence the lump is red, hot to touch and tender. The patient may have signs of shock
- **Richter's hernia**: a knuckle of the bowel wall is caught in a hernia sac compromising its blood supply, but the continuity of the bowel lumen is maintained.

The two commonest types of hernias are inguinal and femoral hernia.

The inguinal canal is a 4-cm-long oblique passage that permits the passage of the spermatic cord or round ligament and the ilioinguinal nerve. The key anatomy is summarized below (walls in bold) **(44)**:

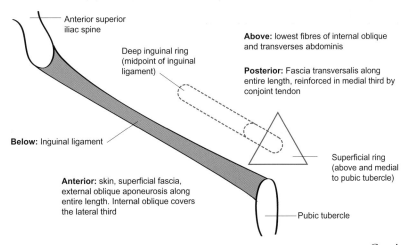

Anterior superior iliac spine

Deep inguinal ring (midpoint of inguinal ligament)

**Above:** lowest fibres of internal oblique and transverses abdominis

**Posterior:** Fascia transversalis along entire length, reinforced in medial third by conjoint tendon

**Below:** Inguinal ligament

Superficial ring (above and medial to pubic tubercle)

**Anterior:** skin, superficial fascia, external oblique aponeurosis along entire length. Internal oblique covers the lateral third

Pubic tubercle

Continued on page 150

Answers
**41.** T F T T F
**42.** F F T F F
**43.** F F T F F
**44.** See explanation

## EXPLANATION: ACUTE ABDOMEN (III)  Cont'd from page 149

Seventy per cent of **inguinal hernias** are indirect, while 30 per cent are direct. There are two peaks in the incidence, at infancy and between the ages of 55 and 85 years. They are more common in males and are more common on the right-hand side.

The differences between indirect and direct hernias are summarized below:

| Indirect inguinal hernia | Direct inguinal hernia |
|---|---|
| The sac passes via the deep ring and is lateral to the inferior epigastric vessels | The sac passes via the posterior wall of the inguinal canal, medial to the inferior epigastric vessels |
| May be congenital | Always acquired |
| Occurs at any age but especially in the young | Usually occurs in the elderly |
| Control by pressure over internal ring | No control by pressure over internal ring |
| Oblique protrusion on coughing | Straight protrusion on coughing |
| Does not reach full size immediately on standing | Reaches full size immediately on standing |
| Descent into the scrotum is common | Descent into the scrotum is rare |
| Strangulation is common | Strangulation is uncommon |

The differential diagnoses are femoral hernia, skin lesions such as epidermoid cyst or fibroma, lymphadenopathy, femoral artery aneurysm, saphena varix, neuroma, ectopic testis and lipoma of the spermatic cord.

The precipitating factors, for example COPD or constipation, should be treated. A truss is indicated for patients who are unfit for surgery. Surgical management can be open or laparoscopic. A herniotomy (excision of hernial sac) or herniorrhaphy (repair of posterior wall defect ± insertion of non-absorbable mesh) is performed.

**Femoral hernias** account for 10 per cent of all hernias and are four times more common in females than males. They are more common in the late middle age and the multiparous. Bilateral hernias occur in 20 per cent of cases.

Femoral hernias have a **high risk of strangulation**, 30–80 per cent present in this manner. The femoral hernias that strangulate are more likely to be the Richter's type. They appear **below and lateral to the pubic tubercle**, unlike inguinal hernias which are **above and medial to the pubic tubercle**.

Surgery is mandatory due to the high risk of strangulation.

COPD, chronic obstructive pulmonary disease

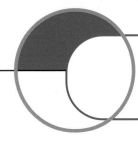

# APPENDIX

## FLUID AND SODIUM HOMEOSTASIS

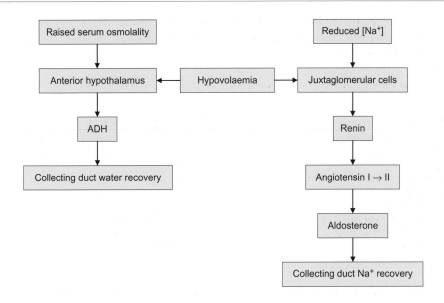

## HOMEOSTATIC MECHANISM CONTROLLING BLOOD PRESSURE

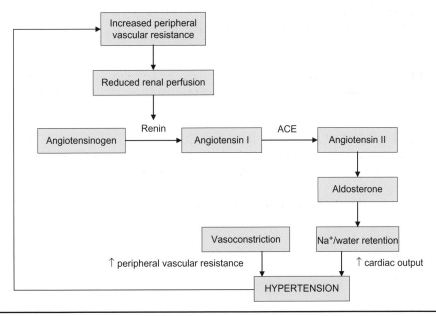

ACE, angiotensin-converting enzyme; ADH, antidiuretic hormone

## BILIRUBIN METABOLISM

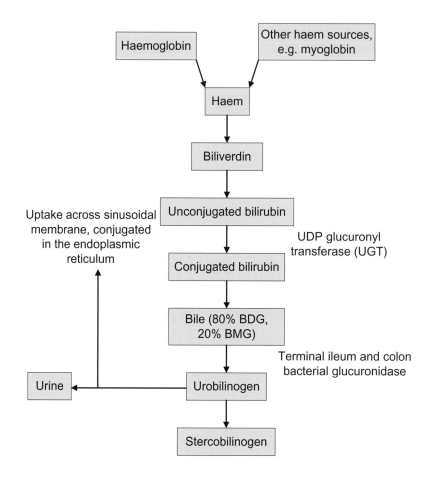

BDG, bilirubin diglucuronide; BMG, bilirubin monoglucuronide; UDP, uridine diphosphate

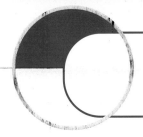

# INDEX